HOW DO ESSENTIAL OILS WORK?

The Science of What Makes Essential Oils So Effective

Keeping it Simple

Dr. Doug Corrigan

Doug Corrigan
Visit my website at www.StarFishScents.com

Printed in the United States of America

First Printing: Aug 2019
StarFishScents

ISBN-9781692094683

Look deep into nature, and then you will understand everything better.

—ALBERT EINSTEIN

About the Author

Dr. Doug Corrigan was led into the world of essential oils by his beautiful but persistent wife, Amy. That first kit was purchased for his wife to keep her from burning down the house with candles, but it eventually transformed their entire family and lifestyle.

Doug has a Ph.D. in Biochemistry and Molecular Biology, a Masters in Physics (concentration in Materials Science), and a Bachelors in Physics with a minor in Electrical Engineering. He started out in his career working with NASA on a series of microgravity research studies that flew aboard the Space Shuttle, as well as with the Department of Energy doing research on new materials. He then switched into the life sciences and launched a biotechnology company that developed novel molecular biology tools that were aimed at helping large pharmaceutical companies discover new drugs faster and more accurately. He is also an avid innovator, and has won over 30 different awards and licenses for his innovations that span from biotech, to nanoscience, to medicine, to energy technologies.

After witnessing the incredible benefits of essential oils being used on his family, Doug had to readapt his entire westernized school of thought to understand the science underlying essential oils. Through his studies, he realized that there is a "theory gap" between western science and natural medicine, and so he developed a model to connect these two disparate worlds. He now uses this model to teach in-depth online video classes that walk a person with no background in science through the basics of biochemistry, molecular biology, and how they relate ultimately to the science of essential oils.

Doug is father to three daughters and one son. In his spare time, Doug loves to compose music on the piano.

You can contact Doug with any questions by emailing DrDougOilScience@gmail.com

You can find more educational content (classes, books) developed by Dr. Doug Corrigan about the science of essential oils at:

www.StarFishScents.com

Acknowledgements

I want to thank by wife, Amy – who has always encouraged me to follow my dreams and to reach for the stars. It's because of her persistence that our family has found the wonderful health benefits of using essential oils.

CONTENTS

PREFACE

Have you ever had an experience using essential oils that made you wonder, "How in the world did that just happen?" I have. Perhaps it wasn't you personally that had this experience, but someone you know or heard about.

Have you wondered if this is just the placebo effect on steroids, or if there is something more substantial that attests to their efficacy?

Is there credible science that explains how they work?

Maybe you are thinking about exploring the world of essential oils, but you don't want to travel too far down the path without understanding the "why" and "how". Or maybe you've been using them for a long time, and now you would like to have a better understanding of how they work to satisfy your own curiosity and to better explain it to others. If that's the case, I think you are going to love the rest of this book.

This book will map out, in simple terms, the science of what makes essential oil molecules so effective. Although my Ph.D. is in Biochemistry and Molecular Biology, this book is written for the non-scientist. So, do not worry - you do not need a science background to understand the content in this book. I designed this book for the non-scientist. That being said, I think any biochemist or other scientist would find this information intriguing. This information is not taught in classes focused on the world view of westernized medicine. For that reason, I believe this book will also be eye opening for scientists are trained in the western paradigm, as I was.

I hope that this tool is helpful to you and the friends, family, and colleagues in your life.

I. INTRODUCTION

Why I Wrote This Book

I f you're reading this book, you are probably considering using essential oils but need to have some more evidence and rationale as to their efficacy and workings. Or, perhaps, you've been using oils for a long time now and you simply have no clue why they work ---you just know from experience that they do, in fact, work, and now you'd like to deepen your understanding. If either of those scenarios describes you, then this is the book for you.

Why did I write this book? Well, being a curious biochemist, I went looking for the "why" in the "consumer" literature and I came up short. I couldn't find a resource that explained the "why." In the essential oil community, there are plenty of great reference books that describe the "what" (i.e., the chemical structures of the oils), and the how (i.e., how to use/apply them), but they all leave out the gap in between --- Why do they work so well? What is it about essential oils that produces their activity? What kind of activity do they possess at the cellular and physiological level? Is there science to prove that they work?

But, volumes upon volumes of research exist in the published peer-reviewed journals about the molecular biology and physiology of essential oils and their constituents. A search of the exact phrase "essential oil" turns up over 8,400 references in PubMed (https://www.ncbi.nlm.nih.gov/pubmed/), and this doesn't include the large number of articles that are essentially about the science of essential oils but that don't use that particular phrase in their title or abstract. There's plenty of research to begin understanding how they work, it's just not being communicated properly to the average user of essential oils. This book aims to fix that. By the way, PubMed and Google Scholar should become your new best friend, if they aren't already.

Because I saw this gap, I began to create educational material that was crafted to teach the average person the answer to the "why" question. I started teaching online courses through social media, and literally thousands and thousands of people were immediately interested and sharing the content with their friends, family, and peers. I received a vast amount of feedback that what I had been creating is exactly what had been missing. I was filling a big need in the essential oil community. I was encouraged to take this information and distill it down into a book that the average person could understand, and that wouldn't put people to sleep like some essential oils have the capacity to do when diffused near the bed at night. Therein lies the challenge --- developing a resource that is simple, but that explains complex concepts to a curious mind. I hope I have created something that teaches you the science in a simple way while keeping you excited about the oils, even if you have no interest in science.

First, a little bit about my background and then a little about how our family started using essential oils. I am a scientist at heart. I started out in Physics. I received my Bachelor's and Master's Degrees in Physics, and performed research for NASA and Oak Ridge National Lab. In my experiences with NASA I was part of a research team that designed material science experiments that flew about the Space Shuttle. These were experiments that focused on understanding the fundamental science of how materials form. I also performed research at the Oak Ridge National Lab (a Department of Energy National Research Lab that now conducts fundamental research) in their physics division on investing the properties of new, crystalline materials.

After these experiences, I decided to change directions in a "major" (pun intended) way. I decided to go back to school and obtain my Ph.D. in Biochemistry and Molecular Biology at the Quillen College of Medicine. I initially thought I should go back to school to become a medical doctor, but my wife quickly reminded me that I pass out at the sight of blood. So, I decided to work with little petri dishes, microscopic molecules, test tubes, and fancy pieces of analytical equipment where blood and guts were nowhere to be found. This was better for the way my brain operated anyway, as I was used to thinking at the molecular level because of my experiences in quantum physics.

This was a new field for me, which made it thoroughly exciting. My goal was to go into a field where I could directly work on scientific research that led to improving people's health. After graduating, and with the help of some great minds, I launched a biotechnology company that engineered novel biotechnology tools for large pharmaceutical companies. The tools that we developed were designed to enable drug companies to discover new drug molecules much faster and with higher accuracy. Also, the tools we created were designed to help researchers develop next-generation drugs that could work against highly infectious drug-resistant viruses that were masters of mutating to evade the drug's effectiveness. It was this experience that really educated me on the western paradigm of pharmaceutical drug discovery. We will discuss some of this in this book, and it will open your eyes to the major differences between the western approach and the natural approach.

After this experience, I began consulting for other high-tech companies who were "stuck" technologically. They needed an invention or an innovation that would help them achieve bringing a new product or process to market. Through these experiences, I have won over 30 awards for different inventions and technologies in a variety of fields, including biotechnology, medicine, nanotechnology, advanced materials, optical materials, electronic devices, and physical rehabilitation technologies, among others. So, science runs through my blood, even though I hate blood. And I bring all of the scientific experience and understanding to the table when I think about and explain how essential oil molecules work.

Truth be told, my beautiful wife, Amy, is the one who brought me into the world of essential oils. So, she's the smarter one. Females always are. The story goes a little something like this: My wife loved to use scented candles around the house. In the fall, the fall candles came out. At Christmas, the Christmas candles came out. And they were EVERYWHERE. The artificial scents gave me a headache, and.... I was very concerned that she was going to burn the house down. I imagined little flickering lights giving off noxious fumes ready to burn the house down as soon as we left one unattended during a small unexpected earthquake (yes, I have some issues with paranoia). A good friend of ours who is a Nurse Practitioner, asked me if I would like to get my wife an essential oil kit from the largest essential oil company in the world as a birthday present. I asked her what they were used for, and she explained their range of uses, including aroma, supporting health, etc.

The only part I heard her say was the aroma part. I was sold. I always have trouble deciding what I should get my wife as a gift, and here was someone handing it to me on a silver platter. The perfect gift. I figured that women like to collect stuff, and this would give her something to collect. There's hundreds of oils, so I figured I could surprise her with a new oil every year. It would be the gift that kept on giving and I would never have to make another agonizing gift decision ever again. For a male, this was a veritable gold mine of brownie points, and getting off the couch and out of the doghouse for years to come. If this was a natural way to get my wife to stop using candles, I was in. I bought her the starter kit for her birthday (which includes a diffuser), and she started diffusing the oils around the house almost immediately.

I noticed a few things. First, I didn't get headaches from the essential oils. There were some I liked more than others, but none of them gave me a headache like the artificial fragrances. Second, I noticed that I felt calm and relaxed when they were being diffused around our house and in our bedroom. The good news was that all of the candles eventually went away as little diffusers took their place.

But, my wife is very keen. She's a smart cookie. With a degree in Biology and always being interested in pursuing a medical career, she was very tuned into researching out health issues for our family. And my wife is the queen of internet research. Whenever she buys a new pen, she researches out every single product online before making a purchasing decision (ok, that's a little bit of an exaggeration, but you get my point). She had gone through the same type of analysis with the different companies that sell essential oils, and she discovered that this particular company was the best in terms of quality, experience, and knowledge. Since we were already using these oils from the kit I had purchased her for her birthday, we were set.

We have four children. Two of them are little girls that we adopted from China. Each of them had their own set of bad health issues. One of our girls was constantly at the doctor's office getting X-rays and medications for issues related to her lungs.

Our other adopted daughter had her own unique set of health problems. My wife, being the researcher that she is, found out what oils were best to use and started diffusing them in their rooms at night, and applying them to their skin. We observed immediate transformations in both girls, and these transformations have persisted for the last several years. If we fail to use the oils for any number of reasons (travel, out of stock, etc), the benefits go away and they revert back within a short period of time.

I was very sceptical at first. Being a product of the western pharmaceutical approach as a researcher made it difficult for me to understand how they were working, or to even believe that they could work. So, I initially brushed this off as a "placebo" effect. But, my wife just kept using them. I figured she wasn't doing any harm, and even if it was a placebo effect, it was doing some good for our girls, so why upset the apple cart?

Then, one day, I had an issue. A small one, but something that would have taken weeks to come to a resolution within my aging body. (I'm 47, and YES I'm a little melodramatic). I applied an essential oil that my wife instantly whipped out of the kitchen drawer for times such as these, and I saw immediate results in a few hours. THIS WAS IMPOSSIBLE!! IS THIS SOME KIND OF VOODOO MAGIC?

At this point, I started studying. I bought books, but I wasn't satisfied because they didn't answer the why. I then delved into the research literature and I found a treasure trove. I thought, "PEOPLE NEED TO KNOW ABOUT THIS!!!" and I began the hard work of creating educational materials to start teaching folks how they work at the molecular level.

And that is how this book got started. It's important to understand that this book will not answer every single question that you have. I need to keep this book short and sweet so that the average person can read it in a short period of time and doesn't feel overwhelmed by detailed science that they may have never been exposed to before. Therefore, I purposefully designed this book to deal with high-level concepts and the basics.

But these are "basics" that I can assure you that most people who are using essential oils have never been exposed to before. The reason is because I teach this material from my experiences and perspective. I present the material with a fresh understanding. If you choose to keep reading, I promise I won't talk about blood and guts, but little tiny molecule-ey and cellular-ly thingies...

So, let's dive in, shall we? Are you curious? Keep reading.

II. WHY I USE ESSENTIAL OILS

My Top 10

Now that our family has used essential oils for quite some time and we can step back and really look at the big picture, I would like to share with you what I believe to be my "top 10" reasons why our family uses essential oils. In parts of this list, you will start to see "hints" as to how essential oil molecules work, which we will dive deeper into in the rest of the book.

1) Replacing Artificial Scents – As mentioned in the introduction, what really motivated my wife and I to start using essential oils was the prospect of replacing the candles in our home which were releasing artificial scents. These scents almost always caused me to immediately develop a headache. When we started diffusing different essential oils in our home rather than burning candles that release artificial scents, my headaches disappeared. The diversity of oils that are available, and the blends thereof, provide an almost limitless variety of aromas that can be produced for any mood or occasion. In addition, a variety of bioactivities can be produced through their activation of the olfactory-limbic system, which controls the areas of the brain involved in memory, emotions, and homeostasis of body functions. Diffusing oils around our home has not only provided our home with a natural means to produce a variety of scents, but it has also provided our family with great emotional and health support through the different oils and blends that are available.

2) Supporting Our Kids' Health – Two of our four children had serious chronic health conditions that required constant observation and appropriate intervention. By using the right combination of oils topically and aromatically in both of our children, immediate benefits were realized. These benefits have continued for five years now consistently. When we stop using these oils, either because of running out, or forgetfulness, these benefits immediately disappear. It's quite obvious from an objective, scientific perspective that the correlation between benefits and essential oil usage is not due to a placebo effect. For this reason, we will continue to use specific oils for our children.

3) Supporting Our Health – What good are healthy children if parents are not functioning in their best state of health? Both my wife and I have used oils to support our health in a variety of specific ways over the last several years. We have enjoyed both immediate and sustained improvement in conditions that are conducive to maintaining and supporting our health. I, for one, have experienced several very dramatic and specific occurrences that couldn't be explained away, and that couldn't have been dealt with in any other "western" manner with any chance of success. These occurrences are what ultimately convinced me that essential oils have quite a considerable range of efficacious activities that can't be mimicked with other more traditional approaches.

4) Safety and Side-Effects – Essential oils enjoy the added benefit of offering these pronounced, distinctive, and potent bioactivities while offering a very attractive safety and side-effect profile. If the doses employed with normal essential oil usage were applied to most drugs, the person using the drugs in this manner would die almost immediately. The list of side-effects for most pharmaceutical drugs are mind-boggling, and in many instances, counterproductive to the indications of the drug itself. This type of frequent and complex side-effect matrix is not observed in essential oils usage, at least not when they are used properly and with common sense. There are some guidelines that you need to be aware of when using essential oils in order to maintain safety to your body; but these guidelines are at least an order of magnitude more lenient than with most drugs.

5) Synergy – Synergy is the phenomenon that occurs when the result of two or more compounds working together is greater than the sum of their individual activities. 1+1=10, or even 0+0=10 are both forms of synergy that are seen with essential oils. Essential oils are complex mixtures of anywhere from 20-300 different constituents, and therefore an almost limitless combination of synergistic interactions are possible. Scientists have discovered and reported on specific examples of synergistic interactions that take place between different constituents, but the body of knowledge regarding these potential synergistic interactions is not close to being complete. Notice that the benefits associated with synergistic bioactivity in naturally derived systems is not possible due to the major *modus operandi* of western medicine, which is built upon the premise of *one* purified compound interacting with a single target in our body. We will discuss this topic in depth in this this book.

6) Test of Time - Essential Oils have stood the test of time and are not "alternative" medicine – Contrary to popular belief in the western world, essential oils are not new or some fad. Essential oils, plant extracts, and herbal preparations have an astonishing and robust history that extends back thousands of years through many ancient cultures. This is the largest clinical trial in the history of mankind -a clinical trial that was performed on millions of people with different nationalities and genetic backgrounds, over thousands of years. Many of these cultures were disconnected in geography and time and, yet, they all converged on the same conclusion: Plants and plant extracts have amazing medicinal qualities. This is well documented in ancient texts, archeology, and other literature. Western medicine is really the new kid on the block, and because it's comparatively young, the long-term effects of western medicine are unknown. Because of this history and more modern research that corroborates their historical benefits, essential oils are part of the European Pharmacopoeia (Ph. Eur.) and are prescribed by medical professional routinely for a variety of conditions. The United States is playing catch-up here, unfortunately.

7) Modern Research Proves Their Benefits – Many people do not realize that there is a significant body of peer-reviewed research, and even clinical trials, that are associated with essential oils. There are literally thousands of articles that one can read to learn more. One has to only sit down at a computer, pull up PubMed or Google Scholar, and type in essential oil and any other search term that they would like to append. I recommend using Google Scholar when performing searches. We will discuss this in detail in a future chapter.

scholar.google.com

8) Health Maintenance – Unfortunately, many Americans are born into the western routine of living recklessly and paying for expensive medical interventions whenever their lifestyle catches up to them. It's always a better practice to introduce routines into your lifestyle that maintain and support your body at optimal health. It makes sense to incorporate some very simple things into our lifestyle now so that we aren't paying the piper later.

9) Current Essential Oil Community – The current community of people who are enjoying the benefits of essential oils is quite large. There are millions of members and this is growing exponentially. Why would this growth be taking place if people were not realizing benefits? You can visit testimonial sites and review thousands upon thousands of different stories regarding the usage of essential oils and their positive effects. Again, this "clinical trial" that was conducted throughout the centuries is still being carried out to the modern day.

10) Removing Toxic Products From Our Homes – Lastly, but not least, essential oils have such an amazing myriad of activities and uses that they have found themselves in many different household products, including cleaners, lotions, makeup, hygienic products, baby products, nutritional supplements, etc. This is all part of movement that is currently building strength around the world to remove toxic chemicals from consumer products. Essential oils provide a great pathway to realizing that goal. Essential oils have the dual impact of imparting their function in the product while supporting our health simultaneously. Essential Oil product lines make it possible to replace every toxic product that is currently lining the shelves and cabinets of millions of consumers.

III. EVIDENCE?

Is There Any Evidence That Essential Oils Work?

I s there any evidence that essential oils actually influence our body to realize positive health outcomes, or is every assertion really just a product of the placebo effect? Being sceptical is a good trait, but that scepticism should not cross over into the world of cynicism when we are presented with data that might challenge some of our preconceived notions. It's important to remember that many of us are products of the western philosophy of medicine. These types of western ideas and approaches have permeated our minds since we were children, so it's understandable that we are resistant to accepting a worldview that challenges our embedded thought processes. Due to confirmation bias, it's difficult to really assess data objectively. This is a known limitation of human psychology. But, if we are aware that this handicap is present, we can actively tame our thought processes to be more objective and rational. This is where I lived, but a number of repeated experiences in the life of my family were sufficient enough to allow me to overcome these inherent biases.

In this chapter, I will briefly describe five pieces of evidence that support the conclusion that the efficacy of essential oils is a real phenomenon.

1) The Volume of Peer-Reviewed Published Research on Essential Oils- A good first step would be to sit down at a computer. First, go to "Google Scholar." Google Scholar searches the world's library of peer-reviewed journal articles, books, and patents, and is more comprehensive than PubMed. However, you can certainly go through this same exercise in PubMed.

scholar.google.com

Type in the phrase "essential oils" in quotations to search for that exact phrase in the title, abstract, or keywords of the papers. That search will return 2 million results. You can also search for "essential oil", and that will return ~500,000 results. Now, not all of these articles will be about the health benefits of essential oils, but you can peruse from page to page and find an endless litany of titles and abstracts of peer-reviewed research papers about essential oils, their mechanism of action, and their documented health benefits. To get more specific, you can search for the following phrases:

"essential oil" bioactivity
"essential oil" clinical
"essential oil" effect
"essential oil" health
"essential oil" properties
"essential oil" (any disease or health condition)

You can also search for the plural form "essential oils" in combination with any of these other key words.

You can also search for "plant extract," but keep in mind that not all plant extracts are considered essential oils. Nonetheless, many of the benefits of plant extracts and essential oils overlap, even when they may be referring to a different extraction method.

This may be the first eye-opening experience for someone to realize that that there may be real science behind essential oils. I encourage you to put this book down, open up your computer, and do the exercise above. Even though I was knee deep in pharmaceutical research, I never imagined this amount of peer-reviewed research was occurring behind the scenes in the scientific community. This type of research, unfortunately, isn't broadcast to the mainstream, and it doesn't make up a large component of the research funds that flow to institutions. Therefore, many scientists are not aware of the full extent of this research. Going through this exercise can be enlightening to the scientist and non-scientist alike.

2) The Track Record and History of Essential Oils – In opposition to what most people in western culture typically assume, essential are not a fad. Essential oils, plant extracts, and herbal preparations have an astonishing and robust history that extends back thousands of years through many ancient cultures. As stated earlier, this is the largest clinical trial in the history of mankind --a clinical trial that was performed on millions of people with different nationalities and genetic backgrounds, over thousands of years. Many of these cultures were disconnected in geography and time and, yet, they all converged on the same conclusion: Plants have amazing medicinal qualities. This is well documented in ancient texts, archeology, and other literature. Egypt (3000 B.C), China (2700 B.C), India (3000-2000 B.C.), Greece (400 B.C.), Rome (1st Century A.D.), Persia (1000 A.D.), Europe (Middle Ages), and France (1800's – Present) all have volumes of texts that describe the medicinal qualities of hundreds upon hundreds of different plant extracts. There are many good books that you can read on this subject if you want to learn more.

This knowledge was not translated into the modern era until scientists, doctors, and chemists in France began formalizing and advancing this knowledge in the practice of "aromatherapy" in the 19th and 20th centuries. These "fathers of aromatherapy" include individuals such as René-Maurice Gattefossé, Jean Valnet, Paul Belaiche, Jean-Claude Lapraz, Daniel Pénoël, and Pierre Franchomme. During the 1800's and 1900's, these pioneers reinvigorated the ancient use of essential oils and plant extracts, and reframed their use into what is now known as aromatherapy. The European Pharmacopoeia (Ph. Eur.) references the prescription of essential oils for certain medical conditions as a standard medical practice, and this is practiced routinely in German and France, with increasing prevalence in the U.K. The U.S. pharmacopoeia is woefully negligent in this area and, in my opinion, requires updating.

In summary, western medicine is the experiment. Natural medicine is tried and true, and there's plenty of documentation to prove that point.

It would be extremely difficult to chalk up the entire body of cumulative knowledge regarding the health benefits of plant extracts to a simple placebo effect. This historical data attests that there is something real that can be repeatedly observed, vetted, and recorded.

3) Plant Molecules Form the Basis of Western Medicine – I would venture to say that most people are unaware that the over 50% of modern drug compounds are molecules that are either directly copied or inspired by molecules that are found in natural products, such as plants.

When western medicine started in the early 1800's with the isolation and identification of singular compounds, the cadre of drugs that resulted were derived primarily from plants. Morphine, Codeine, Atropine, Ephedrine, Quinine, Aspirin, Theobromine, and many others were all derived from natural plant sources. Continuing into the 1900's, and even today, this practice continues. Why? For a variety of reasons, including:

A) Natural compounds are much better at interacting with and binding other natural molecules (like the molecules that make up our bodies) because they are compatible. Naturally derived molecules are more inclined to specifically interact and bind with the shapes that are associated with other natural molecules.

B) There is a symbiotic relationship between certain plants and animals in which plants produce and harbor molecules to sustain and promote health. Therefore, the probability of discovering a molecule in plants that benefits health is much greater than the probability of discovering a drug through screening millions of artificially created molecules designed in a lab.

C) The chemical diversity of molecules in nature is not reproducible by artificial, synthetic means. Many of the chemical structures (i.e., molecular shapes) found in nature are practically impossible to reproduce in a lab. Yet, it is these diverse structures that are needed to design or discover molecules that offer novel bioactivities to treat health conditions.

> *"Chemists started making libraries of hundreds of thousands to millions of compounds. But they were simple compounds. Mother Nature doesn't make simple compounds. Mother Nature wants compounds that fit into particular places." – Dr. David Newman*

A comprehensive study by Dr. David Newman (former director of the Natural Products Division of the National Institutes of Health (NIH)) showed that over a 25-year period from 1981-2006, 52% of the 1,186 new drug molecules developed and approved by the FDA were directly copied or inspired by a natural product. These FDA approved drugs include pain killers, anesthetics, anti-Alzheimer's, antidepressants, anti-allergy, antibacterial, antifungal, anti-inflammatory, antidiabetic, antiviral, and anticancer medications, among many others. We will discuss this in more detail in a subsequent chapter.

Grasp the ramifications of this quote from the Scripps Research Institute in Florida:

> *"Natural products remain the best sources of drugs and drug leads, and this remains true today ....Natural products possess enormous structural and chemical diversity that is unsurpassed by any synthetic libraries. About 40% of the chemical scaffolds found in natural products are absent in today's medicinal chemistry repertoire. Natural products represent the richest source of novel molecular scaffolds and chemistry." – Scripps Research Institute, Florida*

Essential oils are comprised of hundreds of structurally diverse molecules that work together synergistically in our cells. The research of biochemists and molecular biologists has uncovered a microcosm of the interactions that take place between essential oil constituents, and the biomolecules that comprise our cells, as well as the interactions that take place between the constituents and bacteria, fungi, and viruses. The Mechanism of Action (MOA) has been identified at the molecular level for certain constituents, and there is a great deal yet to discover. The bottom line is there is substantial research that connects the way they work at the molecular level to the positive health effects observed at the physiological level.

4) Modern Day Testimonials – There are literally millions of people benefiting from the use of essential oils today. There are millions of families now who are using essential oils regularly in their household. Over the last 2 decades, the growth in aromatherapy has created a very large grass-roots community of millions of people who have testimonies associated with the positive health benefits of using essential oils. Testimonial sites, blogs, and social media groups attempt to capture many of these stories, and the sheer volume and consistency of these testimonials provides strong evidence that the health benefits being observed in our modern era parallel those recorded by ancient cultures.

5) Your Own Story – Personal experiences should not be ignored or downplayed, especially when those experiences can be repeated and are consistent. I have witnessed the benefits of using essential oils for my family, especially my children. Because of my western pharmaceutical background, I was very skeptical that essential oils could provide any sort of efficacy. The effects that I have observed in my family, and myself, over the last five years have erased any doubt whatsoever in my mind that they do, indeed, work very effectively. Some of the occurrences that I witnessed over the years were miraculous by western standards and could not be attributed to a placebo effect due to the nature of the results that I observed. What's your story?

If you don't have a story yet, would you like to make one?

IV. EFFECTIVENESS?

What Makes Essential Oils So Effective?

I f I had to summarize the general categories of properties that explain the effectiveness of essential oil molecules, I would use the categories briefly presented in this chapter. This is a brief description, and we will be exploring these properties in more detail to varying degrees, but this is a good list to have memorized and to be able to describe in your own words.

1) Physiological Bioavailability - The physiological bioavailability of essential oil molecules is extremely high. This means that essential oil molecules are adept at traveling through our circulatory system to reach the various organs and tissues that make up our body. Essential Oil molecules are also able to cross the blood brain barrier and can reach our central nervous system. Also, due to their volatility, the molecules are able to interact with the olfactory receptors in our upper-nasal cavity to stimulate the olfactory-limbic response. We will discuss this in more detail later in this book.

2) Cellular Bioavailability - The cellular bioavailability of essential oil molecules is also pronounced. The molecules are small and lipophilic, which means that they are soluble in lipids/fats. The membrane that surrounds all of our cells consists of a bilayer of lipids, and therefore essential oil molecules can easily "dissolve" into this membrane and diffuse to the inside of the cell. This means that essential oil molecules do not require a specialized receptor to enter into the cell. In addition, many organelles that are inside the cell (nucleus, mitochondria, endoplasmic reticulum, Golgi apparatus, etc.) are also surrounded by lipid membranes. This means that essential oils can effectively permeate the outer cell membrane, and then travel to the inside of various organelles, including the nucleus where genetic material resides. Essential oil molecules also have limited water solubility and can dissolve into the aqueous environment inside the cell cytosol. In brief, essential oil molecules can reach most of our cells and the insides of our cells with relative ease. This is an important point. Drug companies spend billions of dollars modifying the molecular structure of drug molecules to increase their delivery and bioavailability. This property is already built into essential oil molecules.

3) Protein Interaction Diversity – Now that the essential oil molecule is inside the cell, what does it interact with? Proteins. Proteins are the molecular worker bees that carry out all most of the biological functions in our cells. The ability of essential oil molecules to interact with the proteins in our cells is substantial. Essential oil molecules have a vast range of structural and functional diversity in chemical space, imparting them with amazing abilities to bind to, interact with, and modulate the function of the wide array of proteins that control our cells.

Simply put: essential oil molecules come in many different shapes and sizes, which enables them to interact with different proteins, which come in many different shapes in sizes. Think of the proteins like a "lock", and the essential oil molecules like a "key". Since there are many different proteins in our cells, there are many locks, which require many different keys. The different shapes and sizes of essential oil molecules enable them to function as keys. In fact, their chemical novelty and diversity are much greater than the comparatively limited set of molecules that man can synthesize in the lab. For this reason, the pharmaceutical industry still looks to plant molecules to discover new drugs (>50% of new drugs are inspired by natural molecules). This chemical novelty and structural diversity imparts essential oil molecules with a superior ability to interact with a vast array of proteins and to shift the cellular environment back towards homeostasis (equilibrium). We will discuss this in greater detail later in the book.

4) Root Causes Vs. Symptoms – The tendency of essential oil molecules is to deal with deeper, root causes rather than superficial symptoms. We will discuss the reasons why in a future chapter. In brief, since the molecules are small and amazingly diverse in structure, they can interact simultaneously with hundreds to thousands of proteins in the cellular interaction network that controls the functions of our cells. This mass, parallel interaction has the tendency to restore homeostasis or balance to the cell. This is called "polymolecular therapy". Compare this to western medicine which uses the approach of treating symptoms using only 1 molecule that is designed to block one particular protein in our cells. This is called "monomolecular" therapy. Because western medicine is primarily limited to developing molecules that block the activity of a single target in our cells, western medicine tends to deal with alleviating symptoms rather than fixing the root cause. More on this topic later in the book.

5) Synergy – When two or more molecules work together to demonstrate a larger effect than the simple sum of their activities, this is called synergy. We will discuss synergy in a future chapter in more detail. Many examples are known throughout the research literature of synergistic multiplication of existing activities or creation of entirely new functional properties by combining multiple essential oil constituents in different proportions. This is not possible with western medicine because it relies on the activity of one molecule. Notice that synergy, by definition, requires more than one molecule. This is another benefit of polymolecular therapy over monomolecular therapy.

In summary, these five categories of properties of essential oils are responsible for their superior effectiveness:

1) Physiological Bioavailability
2) Cellular Bioavailability
3) Protein Interaction Diversity
4) Root Causes Vs Symptoms
5) Synergy

This short list is an ideal one to memorize. Write it down on a notecard and carry it around with you for discussion. This will help your understanding and your ability to explain the science to others.

V. WHAT ARE ESSENTIAL OILS?

A Brief Look into the Molecules

Why Do Plants Make Essential Oils? Did you know that essential oils are only produced by 5% of plants? There are about 350,000 species of plants; therefore, only 17,500 plants are estimated to produce essential oils, and only 400 of those species are produced commercially.

Essential oils do not travel throughout the vasculature of the plant. Instead, they are contained in secretory cells and cavities that are normally located on the periphery of the plant tissue. They are stored on the periphery of the plant in order to exert maximum effect on invaders and physical dangers that attack from outside the plant.

The function of essential oils can be described in two general categories:

1.   Defense

2. Communication

The plant uses essential oils for biological defense to kill bugs, bacteria, and viruses, and to repel herbivores and pests. Plants also use essential oils for physical defense to protect plant tissue from being exposed to ultraviolet radiation, and to protect against evaporative loss of water.

Also, plants use essential oils to communicate with and attract pollinators at the appropriate time.

So, you can think of essential oils as a plant's defense and communication system. This is helpful because it can be directly related to how the molecules function in our body. Remember:

Defense

Communication

Essential oils are complex, volatile mixtures of certain secondary plant metabolites. Essential oils are considered "secondary" chemistry because they are not involved in the core chemistry of the plant's metabolism (which is focused on building plant tissue, producing, energy, and reproduction). Essential oils are "secondary" in that they provide other benefits to the plant other than those critical primary metabolic functions. These secondary functions include:

1) Repelling herbivores and parasites

2) Killing bacteria, viruses, and other pests

3) Attraction of animals and insect pollinators

4) UV protection

5) Plant wound healing

6) Temperature regulation

7) Reduction of water loss.

Where in the Plant are Essential Oils Produced?

Essential oils do not travel throughout the vasculature of the plant and are not involved in primary metabolism. Essential oils exist in secretary structures that are more or less external to the plant (much like your sweat glands) and are there to help the plant with defense, attraction, and some forms of environmental protection to the elements. As secondary metabolites that exert their primary effects external to the plant or on its surface, essential oils are produced and stored in a variety of different plant secretory structures: Secretory Cells, Secretory Cavities, Secretory Ducts, Epidermal Cells, and Glandular Trichomes.

We will focus on glandular trichomes because they are a very common oil gland from which essential oils are extracted. Glandular trichomes are specialized hairs found on the surface of about 30% of all vascular plants and are responsible for a significant portion of a plant's secondary chemistry.

The storage compartment of glandular trichomes is usually located on the tip of the hair and is part of the glandular cell, or cells, which are metabolically active. Trichomes range in size from a few microns to several centimeters and they exhibit a tremendous species-specific diversity in shape and, therefore, they are often used as diagnostic characteristics for the identification of plant species. Trichomes are mainly found on leaves and stems, but they can also occur, depending on the species, on petals, petioles, peduncles and seeds.

Trichomes can be glandular or non-glandular. It is the glandular trichomes from which some varieties of essential oils are derived. Glandular trichomes are usually multicellular, consisting of differentiated basal, stalk and apical cells.

Glandular trichomes have in common the capacity to produce, store and secrete large amounts of different classes of secondary metabolites. Many of the specialized metabolites that can be found in glandular trichomes have become commercially important as natural pesticides, but also have found use as food additives or pharmaceuticals, and, of course, essential oils.

How Do Plants Synthesize Essential Oils?

Essential oil molecules are synthesized in the plant cell by special enzymes, which are proteins that catalyze chemical reactions that build each of the molecules found in essential oils. There are literally thousands of these different enzymes scattered across the plant kingdom, each specialized to carry out a very specific sub-process that is part of the overall synthetic chain that builds the molecule. As one enzyme does its job, the molecule is passed off to another enzyme to perform another chemical reaction. As the molecule is shuffled around to the different enzymes, it develops into its final structure. Because of the large variety of enzymes, a large array of chemical structures can be built.

As an example: Below is the structure of gamma-Terpinene, which is a common constituent found in many essential oils

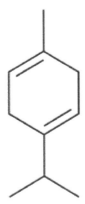

Molecular Structure of gamma -Terpinene

This graphic below is the molecular structure of the protein enzyme that helps synthesize gamma-Terpinene in Thyme. The name of this protein is Gamma-Terpinene Synthase. This protein is not actually "in" the essential oil - it's just the molecular factory that performs the chemical reaction in the plant cell to help make some of the major chemical components found in the essential oil. Essential oil molecules are much smaller than the proteins that synthesize them, as you can see in the graphic below.

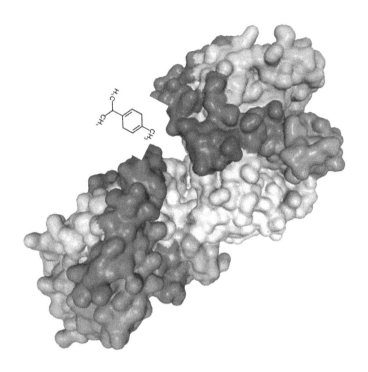

Atomic Structure of Terpinene Synthase, an Enzyme that Catalyzes the Formation of Terpinene in Thyme. The Terpinene Molecule is Shown Alongside the Enzyme for Size Comparison.

How Big Are Essential Oil Molecules?

There are literally thousands of different types molecules that comprise the different types of essential oils that we find on the planet, but they are all about the same size (more or less). And compared to many molecules found in our cells, they are on the lower end of the size-spectrum. In fact, there are not too many molecules in our cells that are smaller than essential oil molecules.

Essential oil molecules are grouped into different sizes. Monoterpenes are a class of molecules that contain 10 Carbons, Sesquiterpenes contain 15 Carbons, Diterpenes contain 20 Carbons, and Triterpenes contain 30 Carbons. The molecular weight of essential oil molecules can range from 150 Atomic Mass Units (AMUs) up to 500 AMUs. On average, they are about the same size as an amino acid. Amino acids are the small molecules in our cells that are strung together to form proteins. Therefore, essential oil molecules are much smaller than proteins.

The image below shows you the relative size of essential oil molecules to some other biological molecules. In this figure, you can see the West Nile Virus, an antibody, and an essential oil. The West Nile Virus is comprised of many different proteins that have assembled into the structure shown, and is about 50 nanometers in diameter, which is 50 billionths of a meter. The antibody is a protein that is about 5 nanometers (10 times smaller than the virus). Essential oils range from 0.8 to a little over 1 nanometer, so about 50 times smaller than a virus particle.

How does this compare to the size of a cell in our body? The average cell in our body us about 50 micrometers, or 50,000 nanometers. So, a cell is 50,000 times bigger than the average essential oil molecule!

Does the fact that the essential oil is relatively small mean that it is ineffective or powerless at exerting its activity to support health?

Absolutely not. Size doesn't matter when it comes to biological potency.

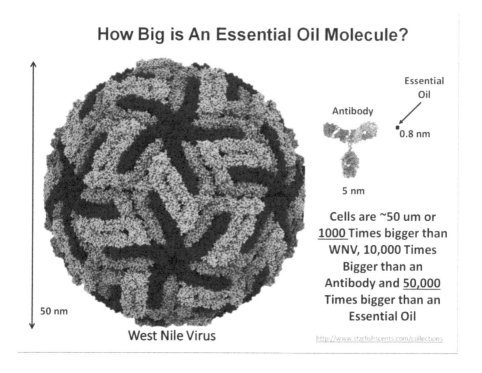

How Big is An Essential Oil Molecule?

Essential Oil

Antibody

0.8 nm

5 nm

Cells are ~50 um or 1000 Times bigger than WNV, 10,000 Times Bigger than an Antibody and 50,000 Times bigger than an Essential Oil

West Nile Virus

50 nm

http://www.starfishscents.com/collections

Size of Essential Oil Molecule Compared to an Antibody and the West Nile Virus.

What's the Difference Between Essential Oils and Vegetable Oils?

Carrier oils are usually vegetable oils derived from the seeds of a plant, and are considered "fixed" oils. Fixed oils consist mainly of mono-, di-, and triglycerides. These molecules have long hydrocarbon fatty acid "tails" and are not very volatile. They are hydrophobic, meaning that they don't like to mix with water, but they are considered larger molecules. Therefore, they feel greasy. Also, the melting point of a carrier oil is much higher than an essential oil's, and they can become very viscous and turn into a solid at temperatures well above freezing.

Essential oil molecules are much smaller. They do not have long hydrophobic, fatty acid tails. They are still hydrophobic, but not as hydrophobic as carrier oils. Because they are smaller, they have a lower boiling point, and are much more volatile, meaning that they tend to evaporate relatively quickly. This molecular difference is what accounts for the greasiness of carrier oils vs the non-greasiness of essential oils.

For this reason, it's beneficial to blend/dilute the essential oil with a carrier oil. The carrier oil can keep the essential oil molecules from evaporating as quickly (especially the smaller EO molecules). So, when you apply the carrier oil to your skin, the EO molecules have more time to absorb into your skin without rapidly evaporating first.

VI. THE DIFFERENCE BETWEEN WESTERN MEDICINE AND NATURAL MEDICINE

Two different schools of thought

I would venture to say that many of us have experienced first-hand how effective essential oils are. If you're anything like me, your first experience with oils may have shocked you into disbelief. Due to my training in the western paradigm of pharmaceutical research and western medicine, this was my initial reaction. Because it was so deeply engrained in my mind, my science brain didn't want to accept what I saw with my eyes. But I eventually came around and began a process of research to understand how these molecules are working at the molecular level.

What helped me to finally grasp the difference was the realization that western medicine is built around monomolecular therapy, while natural medicine is built on polymolecular therapy. Do you understand these differences? This was the key for me. This was the epiphany that unlocked the mystery.

The paradigm of western medicine is based on the premise of one purified drug molecule interacting with one cellular target to impart some type of effect. This is called "monomolecular" therapy. However, in natural medicine, many different molecules are used simultaneously. This is called "polymolecular" therapy. There are fundamental differences between these two approaches.

The first thing to understand is that the cell is a very complex space (UNDERSTATEMENT OF THE YEAR).

If you were to zoom in to a small region inside one cell, the degree of complexity that you would encounter would appear as a swarming universe of biomolecules all interacting with one another. The combination of the different molecules are all interacting, moving, communicating, and influencing one another.

Molecular biologists represent these complex interactions within the cell using an interaction network. What is an interaction network? It's really a simple diagram that shows you what happens when a certain protein or biomolecule participates in an interaction with another protein or biomolecule. That's how everything happens in our cell. Things INTERACT with one another. If you understand all of the interactions, then you understand how the cell works.

You can imagine that this interaction network starts to look like a big interconnected web where you can see the big picture. And from this big web, you can see how interfering with just one protein can ripple throughout the cell in a downstream chain reaction the perturbs the entire network. The network, basically, helps you to answer this question: "If a molecule (a drug, or chemical constituent from an essential oil) interacts with one protein, then what are the downstream effects of that interaction throughout the network? What is the net effect after all is said and done?"

In the diagram below, I show you what the interaction network looks like for just a small set of the proteins in the cell. Each "dot" in the diagram is a particular protein that our cell makes, and each line between dots represents an interaction between two different proteins.

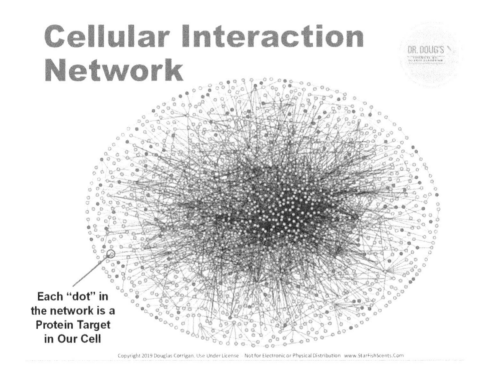

Cellular Interaction Network

Each "dot" in the network is a Protein Target in Our Cell

Cellular Interaction Network in Our Cell

Now, there are over 1 million different proteins, all expressed at different levels within each cell type, along with other complex regulatory molecules, like lipids, ribonucleic acids, peptides, messenger molecules, etc. So, you can imagine that the interaction network for the entire cell is mind-blowingly complex, right? Not even the world's fastest supercomputers can effectively and accurately model this myriad of complex interactions.

To make this easier to wrap our brains around, I'm going to greatly simplify the model. In the graphic below, I show you *one* molecule interacting with a single protein (the top ball) and then a very simple/scaled-down representation of an interaction network. The molecule at the top could be a drug, an artificial chemical, or an individual constituent from a natural medicine, or any other molecule. For the purposes of this example, let's assume that the top molecule is a drug molecule. Each ball in the interaction network is a biomolecule, like a protein, or even a gene within our DNA. The lines between the balls are the communication/interaction that takes place between each biomolecule. Obviously, this is really simplified, but it's going to allow you to see how this all works.

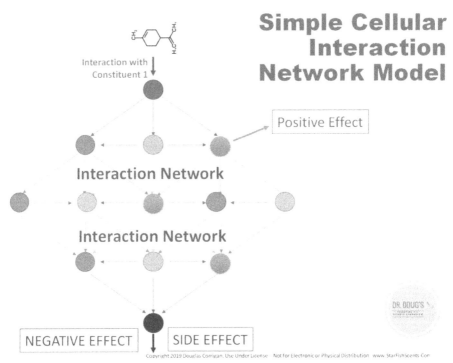

One Molecule Interacting with Cellular Interaction Network

When the drug molecule interacts with the top protein, the immediate downstream effect is something positive. This is almost always the elimination of some symptom, like pain. This positive effect is shown by the arrow on the top right of the diagram.

Let's say that in this example, after the top molecule interacts with the first protein (the top ball), the downstream chain reaction (ripple effect) throughout the entire interaction network results in a net negative effect in our cell. This is shown at the protein represented by the ball at the bottom. Essentially, this one interaction between the chemical and protein causes a negative reaction in our cell after all the downstream ripples throughout the interaction network are taken into account. This is normally called a "side effect." So, for every positive effect (reduction in symptom), there is a corresponding negative effect (side effect). This is almost always the case with monomolecular therapy. With me so far?

Now, let's look at the figure below where I show you what could happen in a scenario where there are *two* different molecules being externally introduced into the cell from some outside source, instead of just one, like the example described above. This is our first glimpse into polymolecular therapy, where more than one molecule is interacting with the cellular interaction network.

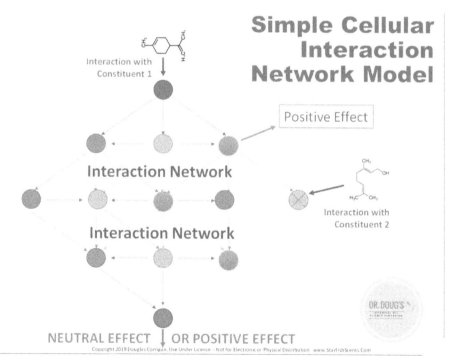

Two Molecules Interacting with Cellular Interaction Network

You can see on the right of the network map where this second molecule interacts with a protein. And in this example, that interaction between the second molecule and the protein basically impedes this protein's ability to transmit the signal from the first chemical throughout the interaction network. You can see the missing lines which represent this effect. When one molecule blocks the effects of another molecule, this is called quenching or antagonism. Molecule 2 is antagonizing or quenching the signaling throughout the network instigated by Molecule 1.

So, in the first example of just one molecule, it was the totality of all signals between the proteins in the network that led to the negative effect. But in this second example with two molecules, all of the signals between the first molecule and the proteins in the network are not being transmitted because a protein in the the interaction network has been quenched. And in this example, you can see that the net effect in the cell is either neutral, or positive. The side effect has either been eliminated or turned into a positive outcome.

What we are beginning to see in this simple model is how one molecule can be deleterious to our body, but when combined with a second, third, fourth, ...n^{th} molecule, how this negative effect can essentially vanish, or even reverse.

So, knowing what we know now, let's answer the question, "How is natural medicine different than western medicine?" In the figure below, I summarize what we have learned to show you the major difference between natural medicine and western medicine.

Mechanism of Action of Natural Products Vs Drug Compounds

- Drug compound MOA: One compound interacting with one cellular target. → monomolecular therapy

- Natural Products MOA: Many compounds interacting with many cellular targets simultaneously.
- → polymolecular therapy

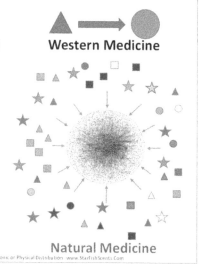

Western Medicine

Natural Medicine

The Difference Between Western Medicine and Natural Medicine

MOA = Mechanism of Action

Westernized pharmaceutical chemistry is built around this paradigm: ONE MOLECULE IS USED TO TREAT A SYMPTOM. This one molecule is designed to interact with one target. This is called monomolecular therapy, and this is shown on the top of the figure above.

But, unfortunately, the one molecule will not "fix" someone's disease. In western medicine, the drug molecule is usually designed to interact with a cellular target to remove the symptoms of the underlying cause of the ailment. For example, if someone is feeling pain due to increased inflammation in the body, then blocking a key enzyme that deals with the pain response does nothing to fix the root cause of the inflammation. It only deals with the resulting pain.

Because Western medicine is built on monomolecular therapy, it is inherently incapacitated to deal with the root cause of an underlying health issue. Monomolecular therapy is more adept at blocking proteins in the cellular interaction network, and therefore, removing symptoms. It's like cutting the wire on your oil pressure light in your dashboard. You still have low oil even though the light is no longer on!

As discussed above, even though a symptom may be temporarily alleviated, there is almost always a corresponding side effect. Because of the nature of how the Cellular Interaction Network transmits signals, an unintended (and unpredictable) side effect is routinely observed with all western medicines. It comes along with the territory of monomolecular therapy.

On the other hand, natural medicine is based on polymolecular therapy, which is comprised of tens to hundreds of different molecules that work together synergistically. This is shown in the bottom diagram in the figure above. The essential oil constituents are represented by different shapes (circles, squares, triangles), and the Cellular Interaction Network is shown in the center. The total effect of these individual molecules interacting with the network has a much higher probability of restoring complete equilibrium and balance to the system than does any single compound. Interactions at many different cellular targets from different directions is more likely to restore homeostasis or order to the system.

As discussed above, the antagonism presented to the cellular interaction network leads to the vanishing of side effects, which is a typical occurrence with essential oils when used at the proper dosages.

Yet, westernized medicine is completely built around using one compound to commandeer this entire network to restore balance. In the Western paradigm, it's more likely that the one compound will shift the network to a new equilibrium that does not match the natural order in the cell, rather than restore it to the correct balance. This altered state that sets the interaction network into a new state of disequilibrium is the primary cause of many unintended side-effects. They are simply unavoidable when you attempt to control such a complex network at one point.

And this same model holds true for nutrition. Any nutrient only exhibits the right bioactivity profile when in the presence of the correct composition of other biomolecules.

If you remember this model and general rule of thumb, the whole subject of health will make a great deal more sense to you.

VII. POLYMOLECULAR THERAPY – THE IMPORTANCE OF EACH MOLECULE

Every constituent matters

I t's important to understand that an essential oil is a complex mixture of anywhere from 20 to 300 different molecular species (also called "chemical constituents"). Because of this chemical diversity, essential oils are considered a form of polymolecular therapy, as we discussed in the last chapter

On the other hand, the cell is comprised of millions of biomolecules that all interact with one another. Molecular biologists represent these complex interactions within the cell using a Cellular Interaction Network. We discussed this in the previous chapter. In the graphic below, I show a highly simplified version of a Cellular Interaction Network.

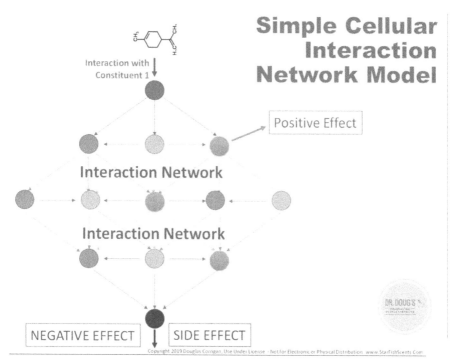

One Molecule Interacting with Cellular Interaction Network

As mentioned in the previous chapter, with one molecule interacting with the first protein (the top ball), the downstream chain reaction (ripple effect) throughout the entire interaction network results in a net negative effect in our cell, or a side effect. Essentially, this one interaction between the chemical and protein causes a negative reaction in our cell after all the downstream ripples throughout the interaction network are taken into account.

As discussed early, when *two* different molecules are externally introduced into the cell from some outside source, the net outcome can drastically change, as shown below.

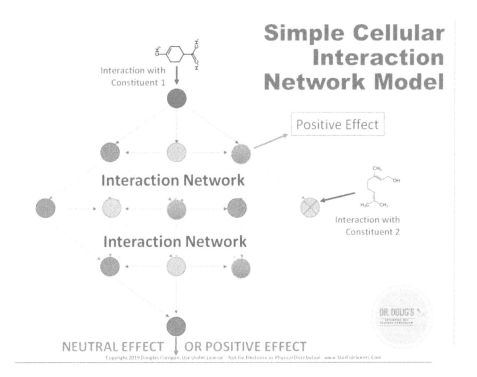

Two Molecules Interacting with Cellular Interaction Network

So, knowing what we know now, let's answer the question, "Do all of the constituents in the essential oil matter?"

Looking at the interaction network, it's easy to see why, right? Let's say a particular essential oil normally consists of 107 different chemical constituents. This is not uncommon. I only showed you two molecules interacting with the interaction network from the outside. Now imagine 107 different molecules. Now imagine a cheap, artificial blend that is just a 3-5 different constituents that have been recombined in a bottle to attempt approximating the natural oil. The effect on the Cellular Interaction Network will look COMPLETELY DIFFERENT! It wouldn't even be close! Those 3-5 compounds will not act the same when extracted from the other 102 compounds.

As you can see from the simple model presented by the Cellular Interaction Network, the combined activities of multiple molecules are not "additive," like in algebra. So, if you have an effect that is generated from 80% of Molecule A mixed with 20% of Molecule B, and you take away Molecule B such that you're only left with Molecule A, the resulting effect may not be close to the same. The effect might completely disappear or change its nature when Molecule B is removed. This can even be the case if the initial effect was due to a mixture of 99.9% A and 0.1% B. This is because each molecule interacts at a different point in the network, which can have unpredictable consequences.

However, the thought process supported by western medicine is much different. Western medicine is built on the notion that things simply "add" up, and that the majority of the observed health effect can be attributed to just one player. So, if a western medicine practitioner were to come across a plant that was known to heal cancer, they would study the plant and attempt to find the one molecule among the tens of thousands that is imparting this activity. They wouldn't stop to think that it could be the activity of 27 different molecules working together as a team that makes this occur. Why? Because this is not the way western medicine practitioners are taught to view the biological universe. Drug companies make their money off of one molecule doing the trick, so this dogma is entrenched into the academic community. I was brought up in this system, and this is the way my brain worked.

Unfortunately, this flawed thought process has bled over to natural medicine practitioners as well. If a natural oil naturally contains 70% limonene and the other 30% is made of 106 different constituents, a large degree of natural practitioners would attempt to purify limonene from the oil, or to only pay attention to the limonene content in quality control assays.

It's not accurate to say, "Well, since the oil is mostly limonene, I'll get the same effect if I just use limonene. That should be close enough."

Unfortunately, this is how many companies think when it comes to essential oils. The faulty logic of western medicine has infected the thought process of natural medicine, unfortunately.

This same line of reasoning tells you why quality and composition matter. Every constituent is important and plays a very important role in the overall interaction network, no matter how minor. In fact, many of the minor, trace components in essential oils either antagonize (neutralize) a negative effect of another component, or synergize (make stronger) an effect of a major component. Sometimes, a minor component will not be able to exert its positive activity without the presence of another minor component. If you buy an oil where the composition is unknown or not created in the right way, then you are dealing with a completely different animal when it comes to its bioactivity profile. It's not enough just to slap "lavender" on the side of bottle. That tells you virtually nothing.

So, if every component and even trace components of the essential oil are critical, then the process used to make the essential oil from the seed, to the growing conditions, to the harvesting methods, to the distillation methods are absolutely critical. Each variable in that chain of events needs to be controlled. If you are using an oil where that process is not controlled, or if there is no visibility into the process because the oils are bought from vendors post-distillation, then you are essentially using an oil where the efficacy is undefined. Two distillates of lavender could produce wildly different biological activities depending on the complete make up of all of the major and minor components.

Every single molecule is important. This is the premise of polymolecular therapy. Remember that. And this is why it's critical to choose the right essential oil company.

VIII. THE MOLECULAR DIFFERENCE BETWEEN DRUGS AND ESSENTIAL OILS

It comes down to diversity and novelty

Why are essential oil molecules so effective at performing their job, especially when compared to artificial molecules designed by man? I this chapter, I'm going to help you understand the primary reasons why they are so effective.

For a molecule to work, it needs to fit into a very specific geometric space inside of another molecule. A glove-tight fit is necessary for an interaction to take place. In the case of essential oils, a particular essential oil molecule needs to fit in the pocket of its target molecule. This target is usually some other protein that our body, a bacterium, or a virus makes as part of its normal composition. When this essential oil molecule interacts with its target by fitting into a certain pocket, it can then cause a downstream effect in our cells. This is how drugs work. This is how all of biochemistry works: one molecule fitting and interacting with another molecule. We discussed how these interactions work inside the overall context of the Cellular Interaction Network in the last couple of chapters.

Many of the targets that essential molecules, drugs, or other molecules fit into are highly complex protein molecules. These proteins have very defined, highly sophisticated geometries with precisely shaped surface topologies. Because these protein molecules are so complicated in geometry, it's very difficult to find another molecule that will precisely fit into a certain cavity or pocket.

Think of a key fitting inside a lock. The essential oil molecule is the key. The target protein is the lock. Now imagine that the key and the lock are very complex 3-dimensional shapes, and you can see how difficult it must be to have one molecule fit into another in the exact way.

This process is so complex that drug companies spend on average $800 million dollars to develop one drug molecule that can fit into one protein. They have libraries with millions of compounds in them, and they search for one that will "sort of" fit. In my former career, I designed assays that were designed to screen these libraries more efficiently. I engineered tools that were designed to make this process more accurate and more efficient.

Now, after a drug company finds a molecule that will "sort of" fit, they get busy with modifying, tweaking, and adjusting the structure of the molecule so that it will really fit. They also modify the molecule to make sure that your body will eventually metabolize and excrete it, and to lessen the potential side effects. This effort to fit a drug molecule into a specific protein target is shown in the figure below.

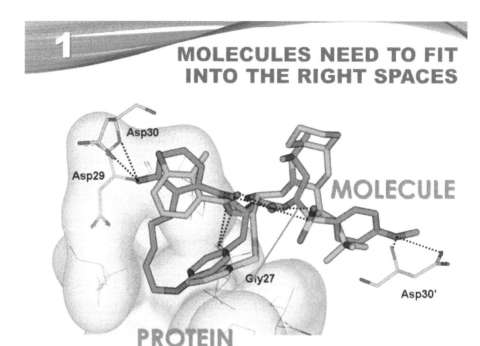

Drug Molecules Fitting into a Protein

You can see in the graphic above that the protein has a pocket with a defined 3-dimesional shape. The drug molecule is designed to "fit" into this pocket.

For example, let's say that you're designing a drug to block inflammation. There's a protein named "Cyclooxygenase (COX)" that is involved in relaying the signals within the cell that cause inflammation. If you can design a drug to block the COX protein, then you can effectively block the progression of inflammation. Therefore, the drug molecule will be designed to fit inside the specific shape of this protein to block its ability to transmit the inflammation signal. Ibuprofen is such a molecule.

Now, here is the key to this entire chapter:

The molecules that humans are capable of designing and synthesizing in the lab are quite limited when compared to the range of molecules that nature produces.

Read that sentence over and over again and embed it in your brain. It's one of the most important things you will learn about natural medicine. In fact, there is an order of magnitude difference between the diversity and complexity of natural chemicals and the molecules that are artificially created in the lab in a beaker. We simply lack the diverse synthetic tools that plants possess to produce the myriad of millions of structures that are possible in what we call "chemical space." Plants produce a complicated repertoire of molecular machines that can morph chemicals into new forms step by step. Many of these chemical structures are virtually impossible to synthesize in the lab.

Therefore, the artificial drug discovery libraries that pharmaceutical companies use to find new drugs are quite limited. Historically, the greatest success in drug development has originated from starting with a naturally copied or inspired product.

The second image below shows you just a sample of some of the diverse structures that exist within an essential oil. These compounds can explore "chemical space" in a way that is unsurpassed by any man-made chemical library. Some of these "shapes" are impossible or very difficult to produce by a chemist in the lab. There are literally tens of thousands of different molecules that plants use to compose the 400 different essential oils that are now commercially available.

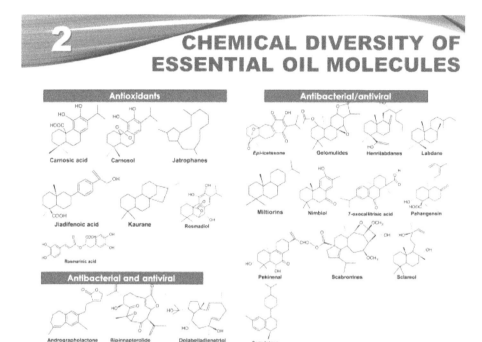

A Sample of Complex Molecules Found in Essential Oils

The image below is a graphical representation of the diversity in chemical space of 192,000 different natural molecules (the gray triangles) and man-made drugs (the black points). The three different axes or dimensions of the graph represent a way of quantifying a particular property of the molecule. It's not important that you understand these three different dimensions of measurement. If a group of molecules are similar in nature, they will tend to cluster together on this 3-dimensional graph. If they are different in nature, they will tend to be spread out on this graph.

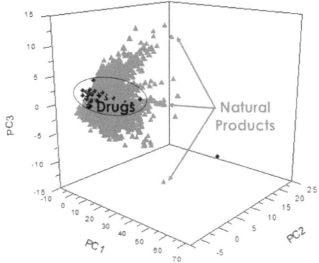

A Graph Representing the Chemical Diversity of Different Molecules

Do you see a difference between the natural molecules and man-made molecules? The man-made molecules are all limited to a very narrow region of chemical space, and the natural molecules span a much larger region in the 3-dimensions of the graph.

What is this telling us?

First, it's telling us that man-made chemicals are boring when compared to natural chemicals.

Second, it's telling us that the chances of one of these man-made molecules fitting into the right space inside of a protein is very small.

That's why it takes pharmaceutical companies $800 million dollars to find one. Why do they go through this trouble when the natural products are so much better at this? Because it's very difficult to protect the patent on a natural molecule. From an intellectual property perspective, it's more advantageous for a pharmaceutical company to own the patent on both the structure of the molecule, and its use. With a natural molecule, they can only patent the use (not the design), and this is only the case if the use of the molecule has never been reported in the literature before. When a pharmaceutical company owns the patent on both the design and the use of the molecule, they can effectively protect their market share on the drug, and gain a monopoly over that drug compound. That's the reason why they are willing to invest the upfront $800 million in research.

But, do drug companies take advantage of natural compounds to "inspire" them? They most certainly do. A comprehensive review by Dr. David Newman showed that over a 25-year period, 53% of new drug molecules developed and approved by the FDA during that period were directly copied or inspired by a natural product.

Listen to what the Scripps Research Institute has to say:

> *"Natural products remain the best sources of drugs and drug leads, and this remains true today despite the fact that many pharmaceutical companies have deemphasized natural products research in favor of HTP screening of combinatorial libraries during the past 2 decades. Natural products possess enormous structural and chemical diversity that is unsurpassed*

by any synthetic libraries. About 40% of the chemical scaffolds found in natural products are absent in today's medicinal chemistry repertoire. Natural products represent the richest source of novel molecular scaffolds and chemistry "
-Scripps Research Institute, Florida

Now listen to what Dr. Newman, former director of the NIH's Natural Products Branch, has to say:

"Chemists started making libraries of hundreds of thousands to millions of compounds. But they were simple compounds. Mother Nature doesn't make simple compounds. Mother Nature wants compounds that fit into particular places."
-Dr. David Newman

From a molecular shape perspective, the bottom line is this: natural molecules are better at fitting into other natural molecules. Man lacks the tools to faithfully recreate the diversity and specificity of these type of unique natural binding interactions. Natural molecules are novel and complex, much more so than anything designed and synthesized in the lab by man.

Benefits of Natural Molecules Compared to Artificial Molecules

Now that we have a good understanding of how the shape of the molecule affects its efficacy, and now that we understand how polymolecular therapy works in the context of the Cellular Interaction Network, let's synthesize this knowledge to develop a list of differentiators that separate the effectiveness of natural molecules from artificially synthesized molecules:

1) **The Largest and Longest Clinical Trial**- The science and art of using natural products for health and medicine goes back thousands of years, with volumes upon volumes of records detailing the benefits and practice. You can think of this as one very large clinical trial involving millions of people from disparate cultures, genetics, and geographies spanning over multiple millennia. In contrast, westernized based drug discovery is the "new comer on the block" as it has only been around for 100 years on a population size that is only a tiny fraction compared to natural medicine; and the totality of its effects on mankind will not become fully apparent for a much longer time.

2) **Molecular Compatibility**- Natural products contain "natural" molecules, and the human body is made up of "natural" molecules. It's more likely that natural compounds will interact functionally at the level of the cell in a more holistic way because of this common thread of molecular compatibility and design. Basically, natural molecules are better at interacting with other natural molecules.

3) **Novelty and Diversity in Chemical Structures** – As discussed above in this chapter, the novelty and diversity of natural molecules in terms of how they occupy "chemical space" is much greater than man-made compounds. In fact, this comparison is not just a simple matter of comparing magnitudes. Natural molecules extend into other dimensions represented in chemical space that are inaccessible to manmade molecules. There are chemical structures found in nature that man finds impossible to synthesize in the lab due to this stark difference. Westernized drug discovery is limited to a relatively

narrow portion of chemical space, which ties back into the second reason.

4) <u>Broad and Diverse Interaction with Cellular Biomolecules</u> – This greater novelty and diversity in chemical space imparts natural molecules with a superior ability to interact functionally with a larger number and diversity of biomolecules that make up our cells.

5) <u>Multifaceted Interaction with Cellular Networks</u> – The diversity in molecular structure imparts natural molecules with the ability to interact with the Cellular Interaction Network at many different points in the network. Compare this to westernized medicine, which is based on the paradigm of designing one molecule that interacts with the network at precisely one target. Targeting the system at one interaction point perturbs the network into a new equilibrium that is unnatural to the cell. This inevitably leads to side-effects. In the polymolecular approach afforded by essential oil molecules, the cellular interaction network is targeted at hundreds of different interaction points. This multifaceted interaction greatly increases the probability and propensity of the natural product to restore balance and homeostasis to the cellular network in a more holistic way through a system of "checks and balances" and counteracting biomolecular interactions. In short, the natural approach leads to:

a) A holistic approach to restoring homeostasis.

b) Absence of side effects.

This is not possible with western medicine.

6) Immune to Drug Resistance and Genetic Variation- The paradigm of "one molecule" interacting at "one point" in the interaction network gives rise to two other problems:

> 1) Drug resistance in the case of antiviral and anti-bacterial agents, and
> 2) Genetic incompatibility or ineffectiveness of drugs based on the person's individual genetic makeup.

Because of the one interaction point with one molecule, it is very easy for the cell or the bacteria to evade the drug response with a simple mutation or a natural genetic variation that is ubiquitous among different individuals. This is why drugs are notorious for working on one person, but not another. Because of this, an entirely new branch of medicine called "personalized medicine" or pharmacogenomics is becoming a hot topic. In personalized medicine, specific drugs will be prescribed to you based on your genetic background. In contrast, the health supporting capacity of natural molecules, being comprised of many different molecules interacting with the network at different points, is much less prone to changes due to mutations or genetic variability.

7) Purity- Manmade drug molecules are never alone. They are mixed with a series of other unnatural products and ingredients, from stabilizers, to time-release chemistry, to bioavailability enhancers, to preservatives. Natural products, if prepared in the right way, are not riddled with these other toxic components.

8) Dealing with The Root Problem- Man-made drugs are normally designed to treat symptoms, rather than root causes that led to the problem. This is because it is easier to design a molecule to inhibit or block a molecule in our cell than it is to design a molecule that restores function. Because of the diversity of structures found in natural mixtures, their compatibility with the natural molecules in our cellular environment, and their ability to attack the interaction network in our cells at multiple locations, natural products have a superior ability to restore health rather than simply block a resulting symptom.

Why Do Pharmaceutical Companies Use Natural Products to Design Drugs?

As mentioned earlier, many of the FDA approved drugs that are prescribed today have been directly inspired by or copied from a compound that is found in nature. This fact is not proclaimed from the housetops by the pharmaceutical industry. It's also not discussed in graduate level education. I think that speaks volumes. For you to become privy to this truth, you basically have to stumble upon it, or become lucky enough to meet someone who shows you this information. But once you see it, it's plain as day.

Why does the pharmaceutic industry look to nature to inspire new drugs? As discussed earlier in this book, there are several reasons:

1) Natural compounds are more apt at tight-binding interactions with other natural molecules because they are compatible with one another.

2) Plants and other natural sources have been designed to produce and harbor molecules to sustain and promote health.

3) The chemical diversity of molecules in nature is not reproducible by artificial, synthetic means. Many of the

molecular scaffolds and chemical structures found in nature are practically impossible to reproduce in a lab. Yet, it is these diverse structures that are needed to design or discover molecules that offer novel bioactivities to treat health conditions.

Just about all of the drugs that were developed during the 19th century were derived from natural sources. You may be surprised by some of these molecules. Again, this is not something that is advertised. Some of these drugs, which many are still in use today, are listed below. The species of plant from which is derived is shown in parenthesis in italics.

- 1805 – Morphine (*Papaver somniferum*). First pharmacologically compound isolated from a plant. (Structure not discovered until 1923).

- Codeine (*Papaver somniferum*) – Analgesic, Cough Suppressant

- Atropine (*Atropa belladonna*) - Anticholinergic

- Caffeine (*Coffea arabica*) – CNS stimulant

- Cocaine (*Erythroxylum coca*) - Local anesthetic

- Ephedrine (*Ephedra species*) -Decongestant, Bronchodilator

- Pilocarpine (*Pilocarpus jaborandi Holmes*) - Parasympathomimetic

- Physostigmine (*Physostigma venenosum*) – Cholinesterase Inhibitor

- Quinine (*Cinchona ledgeriana*)- Antimalarial, antipyretic

- Salicin (*Salix alba*) - Analgesic

- Theobromine (*Theobroma cacao*) – Diuretic, Vasodilator

- Theophylline (*Camellia sinensis*) – Diuretic, Bronchodilator

- Tubocurarine (*Chondodendron tomentosum*) –Muscle Relaxant

Someone might say, "Well, that was the 19th century. What about modern medicine?"

Dr. David Newman is one of the foremost experts on understanding the role that natural products have played in the development of new drug compounds. He was (now retired) the Director of Natural Products Branch, Developmental Therapeutics Program, Division of Cancer Treatment and Diagnosis, at the National Cancer Institute (a subdivision of the National Institutes of Health).

He has published many papers over his career analyzing the number of pharmaceuticals that originated or were inspired by a compound found in nature. In one of his papers, he analyzed the 1,186 drug compounds that were developed over the 25 year period starting in 1981 and ending in 2006, and tabulated the data. The results of his group's analysis showed that 52% of drugs developed during that period were inspired or directly copied from a natural source.

The classes of drugs that were copied or inspired from natural sources during this 25-year period include drugs that possess the following functions, among others:

- Analgesic

- Anesthetic
- Anti-Alzheimer's
- Anti-Parkinsonism
- Anti-allergenic
- Anti-arthritic
- Anti-asthmatic
- Anti-bacterial
- Anti-viral
- Anti-depressant
- Anti-cancer
- Anti-diabetic
- Anti-epileptic
- Anti-psychotic
- Anti-histamine
- Anti-inflammatory
- Anti-hypertensive
- Anti-fungal
- Anti-ulcer
- Anti-obesity
- Hormone Replacement Therapy
- Osteoporosis
- Diuretic
- Immunostimulant
- Immunosuppressant

Listen to this quote from the Scripps Research Institute in Florida:

> *"Natural products remain the best sources of drugs and drug leads, and this remains true today despite the fact that many pharmaceutical companies have deemphasized natural products research in favor of HTP screening of combinatorial libraries during the past 2 decades. From 1940s to date, 131 (74.8%) out of 175 small molecule anticancer drugs are natural product-based/inspired, with 85 (48.6%) being either natural products or derived therefrom. From 1981 to date, 79 (80%) out of 99 small molecule anticancer drugs are natural product-based/inspired, with 53 (53%) being either natural products or derived therefrom. Among the 20 approved small molecule New Chemical Entities (NCEs) in 2010, a half of them are natural products. ....*
> *Natural products possess enormous structural and chemical diversity that is unsurpassed by any synthetic libraries. About 40% of the chemical scaffolds found in natural products are absent in today's medicinal chemistry repertoire.*
> *Natural products represent the richest source of novel molecular scaffolds and chemistry. "*
> *-Scripps Research Institute, Florida*

And Dr. David Newman:

> *"With the advent of artificial screening libraries, drug discovery hit a 24-year low in 2004, with just 25 unique compounds known as new chemical entities introduced that year. The advent of new drug discovery techniques in recent years has*

> *diverted pharmaceutical company resources away from natural sources of new drug compounds.*
>
> *Chemists started making libraries of hundreds of thousands to millions of compounds. But they were simple compounds. Mother Nature doesn't make simple compounds. Mother Nature wants compounds that fit into particular places."*
> *– Dr. David Newman*

As you can see, the pharmaceutical industry is well aware of the advantage of natural molecules, but this point is minimized in their marketing. In addition, this information is not broadcast in the academic community, either at the graduate or research level. It's quite frustrating that this information isn't more readily transparent, and that more credit isn't given to the power of natural molecules to solve health issues.

Essential oils are full of these molecules, and the research around any one of these molecules could fill up multiple dissertations. It's unfortunate that more research money isn't directed towards harnessing the power that is already present in nature.

References

Newman, David J., and Gordon M. Cragg. "Natural products as sources of new drugs over the last 25 years⊥." Journal of natural products 70.3 (2007): 461-477.

Ganesan, A. "The impact of natural products upon modern drug discovery." Current opinion in chemical biology 12.3 (2008): 306-317.

Newman, David J. "Natural products as leads to potential drugs: an old process or the new hope for drug discovery?." Journal of medicinal chemistry 51.9 (2008): 2589-2599.

Dias, Daniel A., Sylvia Urban, and Ute Roessner. "A historical overview of natural products in drug discovery." Metabolites 2.2 (2012): 303-336.

Newman, David J., and Gordon M. Cragg. "Natural products as sources of new drugs over the 30 years from 1981 to 2010." Journal of natural products 75.3 (2012): 311-335.

Cragg, Gordon M., David J. Newman, and Kenneth M. Snader. "Natural products in drug discovery and development." Journal of natural products 60.1 (1997): 52-60.

Newman, David J., Gordon M. Cragg, and Kenneth M. Snader. "The influence of natural products upon drug discovery." Natural product reports 17.3 (2000): 215-234.

Cragg, Gordon M., Paul G. Grothaus, and David J. Newman. "Impact of natural products on developing new anti-cancer agents." Chemical reviews 109.7 (2009): 3012-3043.

IX. THE POWER OF SYNERGY

Sometimes, Zero + Zero equals ten

S ynergy is a very important topic when it comes to essential oils. Synergy is only possible when there is more than one molecule, which is the basis of polymolecular therapy. In Western medicine, which is based on monomolecular therapy, synergy is not possible.

In my opinion, synergy is a misunderstood and misused term. It's one of the most powerful attributes of natural products, but many people rarely understand what it truly means or how it works. This is due to the vestiges of western medicine which have programmed minds to think in terms of monomolecular therapy. By definition, synergy is a foreign concept to monomolecular therapy. Individual drug compounds, which are the hallmark of westernized medicine, cannot elicit synergy.

In simple terms, synergy results when the combination of two or more components results in an effect that is greater than the sum of each component's contribution, or when an entirely new effect is observed that is not present in any of the components individually.

There are different categories of synergy, and the exact number of types will vary depending on who you talk to. I like to define 3 different types of synergy, and I will introduce what I think is a fourth "pseudo" type of synergy in Chapter 11. The figure below illustrates the 3 main types of synergy:

3 Different Types of Synergy

$$1 + 1 = 10$$

combined effect is more than the sum, but it's the same type of effect

$$0 + 0 = 10$$

neither component exhibits effect, but when in combination they do

$$1 + 1 = Z$$

the type of effect is not represented by either

The Three Main Types of Synergy

The first type of synergy is represented by $1 + 1 = 10$. This is where two different chemical constituents (for example, two different constituents in an essential oil) have the same activity. For example, let's say that two constituents both have anti–bacterial activity. For the sake of argument, each constituent has a level of antibacterial activity that we'll define as "1". What happens when both compounds are put together? If synergy wasn't present, then the combination of the two molecules would simply be their sum: 1 =1 = 2.

However, if these two molecules work synergistically, then their net activity could be represented by: 1 + 1 = 10. This is a five-fold synergy, because the sum should have been 2 without synergy.

I think most people are familiar with the first type of synergy, namely that that 1+1=10 is an example of synergy; however, what most people never consider is the example of 0 + 0 = 10. In this second type of synergy, both components have no bioactivity worth mentioning when used in an isolated fashion. Even if you were to use a very high concentration of either component, you would not observe any activity. In the second type of synergy, activity is not realized until they are used together, and only when they are in the company of one another.

How can this be? Let's take a look at the figure below:

Simple Synergy Model

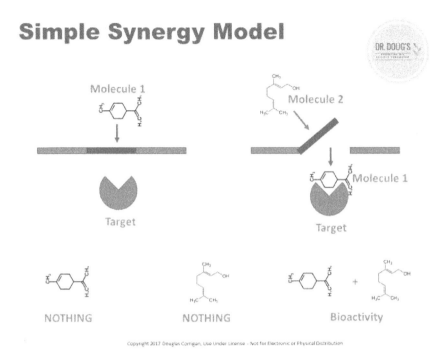

A Simple Synergy Model to Understand the Second Type of Synergy

On the top left of the figure, you see a scenario where an isolated compound needs to go through a "door" in order to exert its activity somewhere else in the cell. This compound has the "potential" to cause an effect when it gets to the "target" sitting on the other side of the door, but it can't get to the target because it doesn't have the "lock" to the door. Regardless of how much of this compound is present, it will never be able to travel through the door. Therefore, it is useless. Its activity is precisely ZERO.

On the top right, you see another scenario where a second, different, molecule comes along. This molecule has the key to the door. However, this molecule is not able to exert any activity because it cannot interact with the target. It can only open the door. Therefore, by itself, this second molecule's activity is also precisely ZERO.

Now, when both molecules are present at the same time, they are able to cooperatively assist one another to cause the desired activity. It's a team effort, and each molecule is necessary to realize the final outcome. Molecule 2 opens the door, while Molecule 1 goes through the door and does its job by interacting with the target on the other side of the door. "Potential" activity has now turned into "actual" activity. Either compound by itself is basically useless. Only when used together can an effect be realized inside the cell.

Notice something? There doesn't have to be a very much of the door-opening molecule around. You just need enough to open the door (tuck away in your mind the term "trace compound"). After the door is opened, increasing the amount of the second molecule will not help. In fact, it may do more harm than good if too much is around.

These first two types of synergy are the reasons why many essential oils are profoundly effective. There are components in the essential oil that occur at a fraction of a percent (these are called trace components). In the western way of thinking, one would think that these trace components are completely useless. "Get rid of them!" shout the western reductionists.

"Reconstitute the oil by combining together only a few of the major components!" is the mantra of the cheap-oil enthusiast. This type of thinking is the result of the western philosophy of medicine. These are the types of thought processes that go through the minds of those who have been trained in the worldview of monomolecular therapy. Because of my training, I used to think like this.

In westernized medicine, one drug molecule is designed to interact with one cellular target. That's it. An entire biological ecosystem has been reduced to a single interaction. And this thought process pervades western thought. If a plant extract consisting of hundreds of components has a few that are the major constituents, then western philosophy would argue that everything else can be thrown away. In fact, western thought would tell you to get rid of everything except for one compound!

Can you predict the result of that philosophy? The end result is that you will lose out on every synergistic interaction! Synergy does not exist in the western vocabulary. For synergy to take place, it takes at least two to tango, and the western paradigm is built around the bioactivity profile of one compound.

For this reason, the quality of the oil is absolutely critical. Most essential oil companies who use synthesized, reconstituted, or adulterated oils -- or "natural" oils that aren't produced in an exact way --are ignoring the entirety of trace components that impart the oil with biological power. Paying attention to every detail during the growth and distillation process is critical to producing an oil with the right makeup of synergistic trace components. Again, it cannot be overemphasized that it matters what company you source your essential oils from.

In the third type of synergy, two components come together to create a new type of effect. For example, when a particular antibacterial constituent and antiviral constituent are used together, they may exhibit an anti-cancer activity (hypothetical example). I do not know of any specific examples of this third type of synergy occurring in essential oils, but my hypothesis is that scientists will one day discover that this is indeed the case.

Below, I list some examples of synergy among constituents that are known in the literature:

Neral + Geranial + Myrcene → potent antibacterial synergy

Citronellal+ Citronellol → potent antibacterial synergy

Eugenol + Thymol + Carvacrol + Cinnamaldehyde → potent antibacterial synergy

Pinene + Thymol + Carvacrol → powerful anti-inflammatory synergy

Linalyl Acetate + Terpineol + Camphor → anti-cancer synergy (more detail below)

Example of Synergy - Power Against Cancer Cells

As an example of synergy, we will discuss the activity of only 3 individual constituents that are found in essential oils - Linalyl acetate, terpineol, and camphor. For this particular study, these 3 constituents were isolated from Lebanese Sage (*Salvia libanotica*) essential oil, but they are also present in other essential oils. In this study, the constituents were incubated with the colon cancer line, HCT-116, individually, as combinations of two, and as all three combined. The cells were measured at 24 hrs. and 48 hrs. The results demonstrated that any individual constituent by itself had virtually no effect on reducing the growth of cancer cells. When used in various combinations of two, a varying degree of moderate inhibition was realized. But when the three were used together, they blocked the growth of colon cancer cells by 65% over a 48-hour period.

To boot, when these same three constituents in various combinations were incubated with non-cancerous intestinal cells, no effect on growth was measured. These constituents were able to differentiate between normal vs. cancerous cells.

How do they work? The study showed that these constituents caused the cancer cells to execute a sophisticated series of programmed biochemical steps to commit suicide! This genetic programming for organized cell death is called apoptosis. It is a common feature of all of our cells, but only activated when absolutely necessary for the survival of the host. The constituents just didn't stop the cells from growing, they actually fooled the cells into initiating the apoptotic program and carrying out their own demise. And this "suicide" signal was the most pronounced when all 3 constituents were used together.

This is a controlled experiment where they tested the various combinations of just 3 constituents. The situation quickly becomes intractably complex when there are hundreds of constituents working together---which is precisely the cause of both the wonder and the mystery of essential oils.

Examples of Synergy - Blends

The best scientific data regarding blends can be found in the German Commission E Monographs. The German Commission E is a scientific advisory board of the German equivalent of the (FDA), formed in 1978. The commission gives scientific expertise for the approval of substances and products previously used in traditional, folk and herbal medicine.

The commission became known beyond Germany in the 1990s for compiling and publishing 380 monographs evaluating the safety and efficacy of herbs for and essential oils for licensed medical prescribing in Germany.

These fixed combinations are required to meet a vigorous set of criteria that include evidence of synergistic effects as well as evidence of the improved safety of the product.

Below is an example of synergistic blends of oils that are approved for medical treatment by this commission:

Anise, Fennel, Caraway → indigestion
Caraway, Fennel → Indigestion
Peppermint, Caraway → Indigestion
Peppermint, Caraway, Fennel → Indigestion
Peppermint, Fennel → Indigestion
Eucalyptus, Pine Needle → Cold related respiratory illness
Camphor, Eucalyptus, Turpentine → Inflammation of the Respiratory Tract

Other good blend data can be ascertained by user guides, desk references, and online usage groups where thousands of people share anecdotal information regarding various blends and their effectiveness. I give some warnings and considerations at the end of this book regarding blends. There is still a great deal of work to do for the research literature to catch up to the degree of knowledge that is present in the essential oil community that was gained through experience.

Example of Synergy – Permeation of Molecules Through The Skin

I've discussed specific examples of synergy with respect to anti-bacterial, anti-viral, anti-cancer, and anti-inflammatory activity of certain essential oil combinations, but now I would like to present to you the example of synergistic activity with respect to permeation of molecules through the skin.

When you apply something to your skin, like an essential oil, the molecules diffuse through the lipid extracellular matrix that surrounds your skin cells and eventually make their way to your capillaries where they are absorbed into your systemic circulation. Each molecule in the essential oil moves through your skin at a different rate, meaning that some of the constituents in the essential oil reach your blood before others. The relative size, shape, and lipid-like character of the molecule ultimately determines how fast it moves through your skin.

In the graph below, I have represented the rate at which different constituents within rose oil permeate your skin. Ten different constituents are shown. First, the experiment was done where the constituents were together in the context of a rose essential oil (the first bar for each constituent). Then, the experiment was conducted where each constituent was isolated and then measured for its ability to permeate the skin all by itself (the second bar for each constituent).

Synergy and Permeation

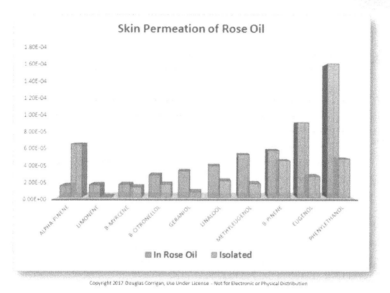

Skin Permeation Rates of Rose Oil Vs. Isolated Constituents

First Bar = in Rose Oil
Second Bar = Isolated

Notice anything? Well first you should notice that for 9 of the 10 constituents, they traveled through the skin at a much faster rate when in the presence of the other partners that make up Rose Oil. When the constituents are isolated, their permeation rates decrease dramatically. This was not the case for alpha-pinene.

Now, if you want to get an idea of how fast the constituents make it into your blood stream overall, you need to weight each of these permeation rates by the relative concentration of each constituent in rose oil. Some of the constituents make up a lot of the rose oil, and some only make up a small percentage. In the graph below, I calculated the weighted average between the two scenarios. You can see that in the presence of their partners, all of the components in Rose Oil will make it into your blood stream about twice as fast compared to if they were each individually applied.

Synergy and Permeation

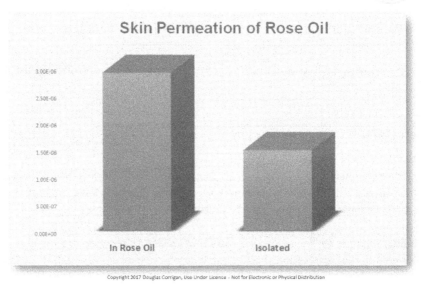

Skin Permeation Rates of Rose Oil – Comparison of Oil Vs. Isolated Constituents

How does this happen? Why does a molecule travel faster when in the presence of the others in the group? Synergy. The molecules work together in a cooperative "team effort" to make each other's jobs easier.

This is why essential oils are being studied as permeation enhancers for drugs and nutrients. If you combine a nutrient or drug with an essential oil, it will permeate your skin tissue much faster than if it was applied by itself. Essential oils increase the bioavailability of many different molecules. This is because of cooperative synergy that exists between the collection of molecules.

And this is why it is important to use essential oils that are natural, and that have the proper constituent profile. If you use a cheap essential oil that's synthetic, reconstituted, adulterated, or not grown and distilled properly, you will lose this synergistic effect.

In Chapter 11, we will look at another type of "pseudo" synergy.

References

Itani W. S., El-Banna S. H., Hassan S. B., Larsson R. L., Gali-Muhtasib A., U H. Anti-colon cancer components from Lebanese sage (Salvia libanotica) essential oil: mechanistic basis. Cancer Biology & Therapy. 2008;7:1765–1773

Schmitt, Sonja, et al. "Variation of in vitro human skin permeation of rose oil between different application sites." Complementary Medicine Research 17.3 (2010): 126–131.

Jiang, Qiudong, et al. "Development of essential oils as skin permeation enhancers: Penetration enhancement effect and mechanism of action." Pharmaceutical biology 55.1 (2017): 1592-1600.

Aggarwal, S., S. Agarwal, and S. Jalhan. "Essential oils as novel human skin penetration enhancer for transdermal drug delivery: a review." Int J Pharm Bio Sci 4.1 (2013): 857-868.

Herman, Anna, and Andrzej P. Herman. "Essential oils and their constituents as skin penetration enhancer for transdermal drug delivery: a review." Journal of Pharmacy and Pharmacology 67.4 (2015): 473-485.

The Complete German Commission E Monographs: Therapeutic Guide to Herbal Medicines. Blumenthal M, Busse WR, Goldberg A, Gruenwald J, Hall T, Riggins CW, et al; eds. 685 pages. Austin, TX: American Botanical Council; 1998.

X. HOW DO ESSENTIAL OILS WORK AT THE MOLECULAR LEVEL

It's all about interactions and pathways

To help you understand how essential oil molecules work at the molecular level, I am going to give you some prototypical examples. By understanding these examples at the molecular, cellular, and physiological level, you will begin to see how essential oil molecules can modulate our bodily functions.

Example 1 – Beta- Caryophyllene

The first example I will use that of Beta-caryophyllene (BCP). BCP is a constituent found in many different essential oils, including Copaiba (BCP is found at highest levels in Copaiba), Ylang-Ylang, Black Pepper, Clove, Rosemary, Cinnamon, Basil, Oregano, and Lavender.

Because of its activity in your body, BCP is in the class of molecules called "phyto-cannabinoids", which are molecules originating in a plant (hence the word "phyto") that activate a class of receptors in the human body termed the cannabinoid receptors. Its chemical structure looks like this:

Molecular Structure of Beta-Caryophyllene (BCP)

You are probably most familiar with the psychoactive phytocannabinoid from Cannabis, tetrahydrocannabinol (THC), that interacts with the CB1 receptor in the central nervous system. Cannabidiol (CBD) is also a phytocannabinoid, but it is non-psychoactive. There are well over 100 different phytocannabinoids found in the *Cannabis sativa* plant.

Beta-caryophyllene (BCP), on the other hand, activates the CB2 receptor, and therefore does not impart any psychoactive effect because it does not activate the CB1 receptor which is mainly expressed throughout the central nervous system.

Humans possess a system termed the "endocannabinoid" system, which is a collection of cell-surface receptors and molecules which activate the receptors. These receptors are spread mostly throughout the central and peripheral nervous system, the skeletal system, organs, as well many of the cells that make up the immune system. They govern physiological processes such as the sensation of pain, appetite, mood, memory, the growth of bone, and various aspects of the immune response. There are two main receptors; CB1 which is mainly expressed in the brain, central nervous system and peripheral organs and tissues; and the CB2 which is primarily expressed in the immune system as well as other tissues. There are also a host of "Orphan" Cannabinoid receptors in addition to these two main receptors.

The CB2 receptor is expressed in the following tissues:

1) Immune system – spleen, tonsils, thymus gland, immune cells (macrophages, monocytes, B–Cells, T–Cells)

2) Brain – not in the same cells types as CB1, and at much lower expression levels. They are primarily expressed in microglia cells in the brain, which are immune cells that provide immune defense to the central nervous system.

3) Gastrointestinal system – mainly supporting the immune response that is attached to the GI system.

4) Peripheral nervous system – in cells that mediate pain.

5) Bone system – osteoblasts (bone building cells), osteoclasts (bone resorption cells) and osteocytes (mature bone cells).

Therefore, as you can see, the CB2 receptor is found in cells that modulate the immune response (anti-inflammatory), regulation of the growth of bone, and to some extent the response to pain.

The CB2 receptor is a protein molecule that spans the cellular membrane. The top of the CB2 receptor is outside of the cell (extracellular) and the bottom of the receptor is inside the cell (intracellular). Shown below is a graphic representation of an immune cell along with the CB2 receptor.

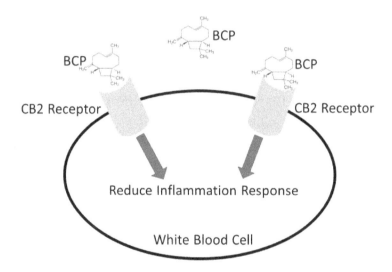

Model of Immune cell with CB2 Receptor and BCP

BCP has been shown to bind to and activate the CB2 receptor. BCP binds to a very specific pocket inside of the receptor and activates the receptor (a molecule which activates a receptor is called an "agonist"). When BCP binds to the BCP receptor, this causes the receptor to initiate a response within the cell.

What happens after beta-caryophyllene (BCP) activates the receptor? Well, researchers have shown that the receptor initiates a cascade of events within the cell through a process known as "signal transduction". Basically, you can think of signal transduction like a race with multiple runners where they hand the baton off to the next runner. Think back again to our Cellular Interaction Network. During this signal cascade in the network, a signal is sent to a particular protein/biomolecule, and then this protein/biomolecule then sends the signal to another protein/biomolecule, so on and so forth. And the signal can begin to branch out to multiple signal partners and become "amplified" in the process. This entire signal transduction cascade is basically a set of instructions that tell the cell how to respond.

Some of the cellular effects of this chain reaction are:
1) Calcium flows into the cell.
2) Potassium flows out of the cell.
3) Gene expression changes (Gene expression refers to a measurement that quantifies the degree to which a given gene is turned on in a cell.)

The net effect is that the immune cells reduce their inflammatory response. Immune cells mediate the inflammation response in the body. When this system becomes overactive in our body due to exposure to toxins, our genetic background, and/or the general health state of our body, a variety of autoimmune and other inflammatory health disorders results, such as

Inflammatory disorders
- Atherosclerosis
- Inflammatory Bowel Disease (IBD) and Colitis
- Rheumatoid Arthritis

- Multiple Sclerosis
- Cancer
- Osteoporosis
- Allergy/Asthma

Indeed, molecules that activate the CB2 receptor have been shown to exhibit anti-inflammatory effects, as well as analgesic (pain relief) effects in the human body. In additional, edema (swelling) can also be minimized due to the fact that edema is one of the byproducts of the inflammatory response. In the gastrointestinal tract, CB2 ligands reduce inflammation and have been investigated as a treatment for colitis. Because of its anti-inflammatory response, the CB2 receptor has investigated as a potential target to treat atherosclerosis and rheumatoid arthritis. It's expression and involvement in the bone generation has brought focus onto CB2 receptors as a target for osteoporosis. Because activation of the CB2 receptor does not elicit the psychoactive side effects that are normally associated with CB1 receptor activation, the CB2 receptor is high on the list of targets for pharmaceutical companies to develop drugs which preferentially activate this receptor for the treatment of a wide variety of conditions.

You have now learned your first lesson on how a specific essential oil constituent works at the molecular, cellular, and physiological level. Keep in mind that every single one of the tens of thousands of different constituents found in the universe of essential oils possess a unique mechanism of action, and the example shown above is just one.

References

Gertsch, Jürg, et al. "Beta-caryophyllene is a dietary cannabinoid." Proceedings of the National Academy of Sciences 105.26 (2008): 9099-9104.

Glass, Michelle, et al. "One for the price of two... are bivalent ligands targeting cannabinoid receptor dimers capable of simultaneously binding to both receptors?." Trends in pharmacological sciences 37.5 (2016): 353-363.

Mackie, Ken. "Cannabinoid receptors as therapeutic targets." Annu. Rev. Pharmacol. Toxicol. 46 (2006): 101-122.
Shoemaker JL, Buckle MB,Mayeux PR, Prather PL (2005) Agonist-directed trafficking of response by endocannabinoids acting at CB2 receptors. J Pharmacol Exp Ther 315:828–838.

Klein, Thomas W. "Cannabinoid-based drugs as anti-inflammatory therapeutics." Nature reviews. Immunology 5.5 (2005): 400.

Klegeris A, Bissonnette CJ, McGeer PL (2003) Reduction of human monocytic cell neurotoxicity and cytokine secretion by ligands of the cannabinoid-type CB2 receptor. Br J Pharmacol 139:775–786.

Cho JY, et al. (2007) Amelioration of dextran sulfate sodium-induced colitis in mice by oral administration of beta-caryophyllene, a sesquiterpene. Life Sci 80:932–939.

Thuru X, et al. (2007) Cannabinoid receptor 2 is required for homeostatic control of intestinal inflammation. 17th Annual Symposium on the Cannabinoids (International Cannabinoid Research Society, Burlington, VT), p 19.

Ibrahim MM, et al. (2005) CB2 cannabinoid receptor activation produces antinociception by stimulating peripheral release of endogenous opioids. Proc Natl Acad Sci USA 102:3093–3098

Steffens S, et al. (2005) Low dose oral cannabinoid therapy reduces progression of atherosclerosis in mice. Nature 434:782–786.

Karsak M, et al. (2007) Attenuation of allergic contact dermatitis through the endocannabinoid system. Science 316:1494–1497

Kimball ES, Schneider CR, Wallace NH, Hornby PJ (2006) Agonists of cannabinoid receptor 1 and 2 inhibit experimental colitis induced by oil of mustard and by dextran sulfate sodium. Am J Physiol Gastrointest Liver Physiol 291:G364–371.

Ofek O, et al. (2006) Peripheral cannabinoid receptor, CB2, regulates bone mass. Proc Natl Acad Sci USA 103:696–701.

Example 2 - Eugenol

The second example is a constituent known as Eugenol. In this example, I will show you how an essential molecule can have a long list of actions. Many times, the bioactivity of the molecule is known, but the exact mechanism of action is not fully understood. Also, many essential oil constituents may interact with more than one protein in our cells. Therefore, a constituent can have many different mechanisms of action. Eugenol is an example of a molecule that has more than one mechanism of action.

Eugenol is a major constituent found in essential oils. It is classified as a phenylpropanoid. There are 3 basic class of molecules that generally make up essential oils:

1) Terpenoids
2) Phenylpropanoids (Eugenol is a member of this group)
3) Hydrocarbons

Phenylpropanoids are named as such because they are basically a 6-carbon phenyl ring connected to a 3-carbon propene group.

Cinnamic acid is an example of a phenylpropanoid:

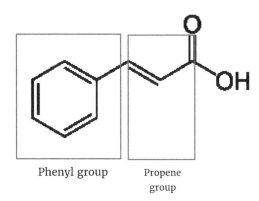

Phenyl group   Propene group

Cinnamic Acid – A Phenylpropanoid

This class of molecules, just like the terpenes, can be modified with different oxygen-bearing functional groups (carboxylic acids, aldehydes, alcohols, ketones, esters, etc). For example, in the cinnamic acid molecule above, you can see the carboxylic acid group on the right end of the molecule. The propene chain can also loop back and cause a ring structure (giving two rings), and two phenylpropenes can link together in different ways. Therefore, there are thousands of molecules that can be derived from this basic structural class of molecules.

Eugenol is a member of the phenylpropanoid class and is commonly found in essential oils in varying concentrations. Eugenol is found in Clove, Cinnamon, Basil, Nutmeg, and other essential oils in lower concentrations. Eugenol has the following structure:

Chemical Structure of the Phenylpropanoid, Eugenol

What can eugenol do in our bodies? Here is a list of documented effects that have been reported in the literature, and the mechanism of action when known:

1) Antiseptic – An antiseptic is a molecule that can be used to block the possibility of an infection.
2) Anesthetic – Antinociceptive – Eugenol has the ability to impart a painkilling effect in a local region of the body.
3) Antibacterial Agent – Eugenol can block the growth of a wide variety of gram-negative and gram-positive bacteria. The prevailing hypothesis regarding Eugenol's antibacterial power is based on the model that eugenol preferentially disrupts the membrane that surrounds and protects the bacteria.
4) Killing Oral Bacteria – By itself, Eugenol can kill oral-bacteria. In combination with other constituents like cinnamaldehyde, thymol, and carvacrol, Eugenol can impart a synergistic antibacterial activity against 7 different microorganisms commonly found in the oral cavity.
5) Eugenol inhibits the growth of Salmonella typhi by disrupting the cellular membrane.

6) Eugenol blocks the growth of Helicobacter pylori, which is the major cause of ulcer formation.

7) Eugenol blocks the growth of bacteria that typically cause the spoilage of food (*E.coli, S.aureus, B.cereus, L.monocytogenes-Lysteria*)

8) Eugenol blocks the growth of a bacteria that can cause urinary tract infections and kidney stones. (*Proteus mirabalis*)

9) Eugenol can even block the growth of bacteria that are resistant to antibiotics. (*Escherichia coli, Klebsiella pneumoniae*). Eugenol more than likely binds directly to the Extended-Spectrum-Beta-Lactamase (ESBL) proteins which cause drug resistance.

10) Antifungal agent – The growth of the fungus *Aspergillus flavus* is blocked by Eugenol, as is the release of its toxin, aflatoxin.

11) Anti-inflammatory – Eugenol has anti-inflammatory activity. Inflammation can turn into a chronic process that is involved in the development of many chronic health conditions. By downregulating the the cyclooxygenase enzyme (COX) enzyme, the production of the inflammatory prostaglandin E2 is reduced. Prostaglandins are a family of lipid molecules produced from arachidonic acid that are used in cellular communication, including the communication associated with the inflammatory response. In addition, Eugenol has been shown to inhibit 5-lipoxygenase activity and leukotriene-C4, another inflammatory pathway in cells. The production of Nitric oxide (NO) in response to inflammatory stimuli has also been shown to be inhibited by Eugenol. Therefore, Eugenol can block inflammation from a number of different pathways.

12) Antiviral – Eugenol can block the replication of Herpes simplex virus (HSV-1 and HSV-2)

13) Anticancer – Eugenol has been shown to be a potent inhibitor of the growth of melanoma cells through two pathways: Inhibition of E2F1 transcriptional activity; and, induction of programmed cell death (apoptosis). In rat models of gastric cancer, Eugenol can elicit anti-cancer activity by blocking cell proliferation through the NF-κB pathway, and by inducing cell-death through apoptosis. In addition, Eugenol can block tumor invasion and angiogenesis, meaning that it can block tumors from developing a blood supply. Also, studies in mice have shown that eugenol can function as a chemo-preventative, as it can inhibit the formation of tumors. In a human colon cancer cell line, Eugenol demonstrated pro-apoptotic activity.

14) Antioxidant Activity – Eugenol can act as an antioxidant that by blocking lipid oxidation. Eugenol accomplishes this by inhibiting the generation of Reactive Oxygen Species (ROS) that lead to oxidation of lipids and other biomolecules in cells. Eugenol can inhibit the generation of the superoxide anion and of hydroxyl radicals (OH*).

15) Anti-arthritic – Eugenol can suppress the symptoms of arthritis by lowering markers in a mouse model of rheumatoid arthritis. Eugenol blocked the infiltration of mononuclear cells into the knee joints of arthritic mice. In ankle joints, it was shown that Eugenol lowers the levels of inflammatory cytokines, such a tumor necrosis factor (TNF)-α, interferon (IFN)-γ and tumor growth factor (TGF)-β.

As you can see, Eugenol is extremely versatile in the role it plays to improve health. Other phenylpropanoids of similar structure found in essential oils can also exhibit different profiles of activity with respect to the above list. Synergistic interactions can also take effect when multiple phenylpropanoids are used in combination.

The two examples given above represent only two constituents found in essential oils. A typical essential oil can possess up to 300 different constituents. Also consider that if you look at the unique identify of constituents that are found across the universe of essential oils, there are tens of thousands of different unique chemical structures. As you can see, if we were to study each constituent in an essential oil and all of the particular interactions they have in the cell, this book would consist of millions of pages, and that would just be the beginning. However, these examples help to provide you with the concepts of how these molecules work at the molecular level so that you can have an appreciation of their complex range of functions and the molecular basis for their action. These examples also help to arm you with some specific examples to discuss with others who may not realize that there is scientific credibility to the use of essential oils.

References

Didry, Nicole, Luc Dubreuil, and Madeleine Pinkas. "Activity of thymol, carvacrol, cinnamaldehyde and eugenol on oral bacteria." Pharmaceutica Acta Helvetiae 69.1 (1994): 25-28.

Mahmoud, A-LE. "Antifungal action and antiaflatoxigenic properties of some essential oil constituents." Letters in Applied Microbiology 19.2 (1994): 110-113.

Chami, N., et al. "Antifungal treatment with carvacrol and eugenol of oral candidiasis in immunosuppressed rats." Brazilian Journal of Infectious Diseases 8.3 (2004): 217-226.

Devi, K. Pandima, et al. "Eugenol acts as an antibacterial agent against Salmonella typhi by disrupting the cellular membrane." Journal of ethnopharmacology 130.1 (2010): 107-115.

Ali, Shaik Mahaboob, et al. "Antimicrobial activities of Eugenol and Cinnamaldehyde against the human gastric pathogen Helicobacter pylori." Annals of clinical microbiology and antimicrobials 4.1 (2005): 20.

Tippayatum, Panitee, and Vanee Chonhenchob. "Antibacterial activities of thymol, eugenol and nisin against some food spoilage bacteria." Nat Sci 41 (2007): 319-23.

Oyedemi, S. O., et al. "The proposed mechanism of bactericidal action of eugenol,∝-terpineol and g-terpinene against Listeria monocytogenes, Streptococcus pyogenes, Proteus vulgaris and Escherichia coli." African Journal of Biotechnology 8.7 (2009).

Devi, K. Pandima, et al. "Eugenol alters the integrity of cell membrane and acts against the nosocomial pathogen Proteus mirabilis." Archives of pharmacal research 36.3 (2013): 282-292.

Dhara, Lena, and Anusri Tripathi. "Antimicrobial activity of eugenol and cinnamaldehyde against extended spectrum beta lactamase producing enterobacteriaceae by in vitro and molecular docking analysis." European Journal of Integrative Medicine 5.6 (2013): 527-536.

Daniel, Apparecido N., et al. "Anti-inflammatory and antinociceptive activities A of eugenol essential oil in experimental animal models." Revista Brasileira de Farmacognosia 19.1B (2009): 212-217.

Kurian, R., et al. "Effect of eugenol on animal models of nociception." Indian Journal of Pharmacology 38.5 (2006): 341.

Bachiega, Tatiana Fernanda, et al. "eugenol in noncytotoxic concentrations exert immunomodulatory/anti-inflammatory action on cytokine production by murine macrophages." Journal of Pharmacy and Pharmacology 64.4 (2012): 610-616.

Kim, Sun Suk, et al. "Eugenol suppresses cyclooxygenase-2 expression in lipopolysaccharide-stimulated mouse macrophage RAW264. 7 cells." Life sciences 73.3 (2003): 337-348.

Benencia, F., and M. C. Courreges. "In vitro and in vivo activity of eugenol on human herpesvirus." Phytotherapy research 14.7 (2000): 495-500.

Ghosh, Rita, et al. "Eugenol causes melanoma growth suppression through inhibition of E2F1 transcriptional activity." Journal of Biological Chemistry 280.7 (2005): 5812-5819.

Sukumaran, K., M. C. Unnikrishnan, and R. Kuttan. "Inhibition of tumour promotion in mice by eugenol." Indian journal of physiology and pharmacology 38.4 (1994): 306-308.

Kaur, Gurpreet, Mohammad Athar, and M. Sarwar Alam. "Eugenol precludes cutaneous chemical carcinogenesis in mouse by preventing oxidative stress and inflammation and by inducing apoptosis." Molecular carcinogenesis 49.3 (2010): 290-301.

Manikandan, P., et al. "Eugenol inhibits cell proliferation via NF-κB suppression in a rat model of gastric carcinogenesis induced by MNNG." Investigational new drugs 29.1 (2011): 110-117.

Manikandan, Palrasu, et al. "Eugenol induces apoptosis and inhibits invasion and angiogenesis in a rat model of gastric carcinogenesis induced by MNNG." Life sciences 86.25 (2010): 936-941.

Jaganathan, Saravana Kumar, et al. "Apoptotic effect of eugenol in human colon cancer cell lines." Cell biology international 35.6 (2011): 607-615.

Ogata, Masahiro, et al. "Antioxidant activity of eugenol and related monomeric and dimeric compounds." Chemical and Pharmaceutical Bulletin 48.10 (2000): 1467-1469.

Raghavenra, H., et al. "Eugenol—inhibits 5-lipoxygenase activity and leukotriene-C4 in human PMNL cells." Prostaglandins, Leukotrienes and Essential Fatty Acids 74.1 (2006): 23-27.

Lee, Ya-Yun, et al. "Eugenol suppressed the expression of lipopolysaccharide-induced proinflammatory mediators in human macrophages." Journal of endodontics 33.6 (2007): 698-702.

Grespan, Renata, et al. "Anti-arthritic effect of eugenol on collagen-induced arthritis experimental model." Biological and Pharmaceutical Bulletin 35.10 (2012): 1818-1820.

Reddy, A. Ch Pulla, and Belur R. Lokesh. "Studies on the inhibitory effects of curcumin and eugenol on the formation of reactive oxygen species and the oxidation of ferrous iron." Molecular and cellular biochemistry 137.1 (1994): 1-8.

LI, Weihua, et al. "Inhibitory action of eugenol compounds on the production of nitric oxide in RAW264. 7 macrophages." Biomedical Research 27.2 (2006): 69-74.

Ito, Masae, Keiko Murakami, and Masataka Yoshino. "Antioxidant action of eugenol compounds: role of metal ion in the inhibition of lipid peroxidation." Food and Chemical Toxicology 43.3 (2005): 461-466.

XI. DEALING WITH THE ROOT CAUSE

Another type of synergy

There is another type of "synergy" that isn't based on amplifying the collective effects of a group of molecules. It's not technically a form of synergy, but I like to lump it into this category because it is based on the collective action of a group of players to ensure that all bases are being covered. So, in this book I'm considering it a fourth type of synergy.

This other form of synergy is based on "divide and conquer," meaning that each molecule affects a different pathway that could lead to the same disease condition or symptom. In reality, any disease, health condition, or symptom can be the result of a wide array of different root causes. In fact, the number of causes and pathways involved in an altered state of health can be in the thousands. This makes it very difficult, if not impossible, for western medicine to deal with the root cause of the issue. If every patient has a unique cause to their problem, then how can one molecule address all possible causes? This is impossible. This is one of the reasons why western medicine is relegated to working downstream of the problem and blocking the symptom. This concept is shown in the graphic below:

Synergy and Overall Efficacy

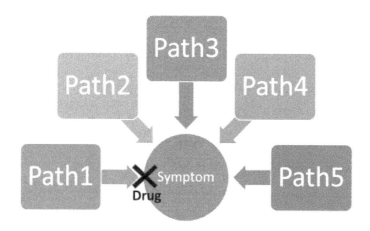

Drugs Block Pathways Closest to the Symptom

As you can see from the diagram, although the drug is blocking the symptom from one pathway, there are four other pathways that could be leading to that symptom in the patient.

As a specific example, there are many different cellular pathways in the Cellular Interaction Network that can be involved in activating the inflammatory response in our immune cells. There are literally hundreds of pathways, if not thousands, that can lead to inflammation. Therefore, there could be many different root causes of why someone might be in a state of chronic inflammation.

However, western medicine is not equipped with the right molecular tools to deal with the plethora of different pathways that could be causing the problem.

However, since natural medicine is based on polymolecular therapy (many molecules), natural medicine is adept at interfering with many pathways that could be at the root cause of the health issue. This is demonstrated in the graphic below:

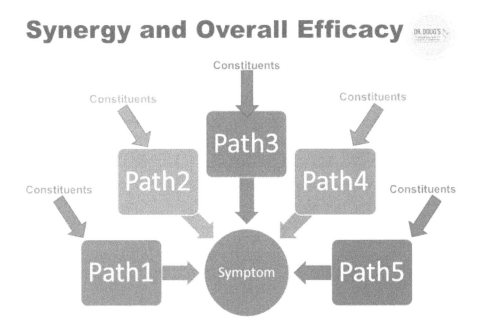

Essential Oil Molecules Can Interfere with Many Pathways Closer to the Root Cause

To provide a specific example, let's take a look at inflammation. There are literally thousands of pathways that can lead to inflammation. The immune system is extremely complex, and a great deal of triggers, both environmental and genetic, can instigate an inflammatory pathway, of which there are many. This being the case, how can western medicine's "One-Molecule-Fits-All" philosophy hope to deal with such a diversity of root causes?

Now, let's take a look at the polymolecular approach afforded by essential oil constituents.

First of all, any one constituent can interact with more than one pathway. We saw this in the example of Eugenol in the previous chapter. Secondly, a combination of different constituents (which is the definition of an essential oil), can obviously affect multiple pathways. The table below shows you a list of some anti-inflammatory constituents and the inflammatory pathways that they modulate.

Anti-inflammatory Activity of Constituents

Constituent	Mechanism
α-humulene	reduction of PGE2, iNOS, and COX-2, reduction of tumor necrosis factor-α (TNFα) and interleukin-1β (IL-1β) generation
Beta-caryophyllene	reduction of PGE2, iNOS, and COX-2, reduction of tumor necrosis factor-α (TNFα) generation. Binding of CB2 receptor in immune cells; Reduction of Nitric Oxide (NO) production
trans-Cinnamaldehyde	Reduction of Nitric Oxide (NO) production, Reduce COX-2, Reduction of PGE2, Reduction of NF-κB, Inhibition of IL-1B, IL-6, Reduction of TNFα, Blocks release of ROS, reduces mRNA of iNOS,
caryophyllene oxide	Reduction of Nitric Oxide (NO) production, Reduction of PGE2
L-borneol	Reduction of Nitric Oxide (NO) production
L-bornyl acetate	Reduction of Nitric Oxide (NO) production, Reduction of PGE2
E-nerolidol	Reduction of Nitric Oxide (NO) production
cinnamyl acetate	Reduction of Nitric Oxide (NO) production
thymol	Reduction of COX-1 and COX-2 Activity, reduction of edema,
carvacrol	reduction of edema, reduction of leokocyte migration
2'-hydroxycinnamaldehyde	Reduce NO, Reduce COX-2, Reduce TNFα
eugenol and isoeugenol	Reduce COX-2, Reduce PGE2, Reduce NO and iNOS
methyleugenol	Inhibit NO and iNOS, Reduce IL-1B, IL-6, and TNFα,
myristicin	Suppression of NO, IL-6, IL-10,
elimicin	Inhibition of 5-LOX
Asarone	Inhibition of COX-1 and COX-2
Anethole	Reduce NO, Reduce PGE2, Reduce number of inflammatory cells, Reduce MMP-9, Reduce TNFα,
Acetyl-11-keto-beta-boswellic acid (AKBA)	Inhibits 5-LOX and luekotrienes
Limonene	Reduces ROS, Reduces NO production, Reduce Monocyte Chemoattractant Protein (MCP-1), Inhibits cell chemotaxis, Reduces NF-KB, Reduces IL-1B, Reduces MMP-1 and MMP-13
Myrcene	Reduces NO Production, Reduces NF-KB, Reduces iNOS, Reduces MMP-1 and MMP-13,

These are just some examples of anti-inflammatory activity, and this is by no means exhaustive treatise on the subject. In fact, there's a great deal more research needed to close the gap between what we know now and being comprehensive.

Essential Oils that are derived from a single species of plant (i.e., a "single), can possess a myriad of molecules with anti-inflammatory activity. Also, blends can increase the number of active players in the mix.

Because we are unaware of the inflammatory pathway that might be causing our issue, it's wise to employ a multi-faceted approach. This multi-faceted approach also enables you to reach further back into multiple pathways to deal with the root cause of the issue, or somewhere along the pathway that is closer to the root cause.

Therefore, the use of essential oils provides a means to deal with the deeper root cause of an underlying health issue, and not just the superficial symptom. This is possible because essential oils are comprised of many different molecules that can interact with various players in the Cellular Interaction Network simultaneously. This is another fortunate form of "synergy" that comes along for the ride when using essential oils.

XII. ESSENTIAL OILS AND OUR BODY

What happens to the molecules when they enter our body?

Pharmacokinetics (PK) is the study of the absorption, distribution, metabolism, and elimination of molecules that enter the body. PK answers the questions: Where do they go? How fast do they get there and in what concentration? What happens to the molecules? What is their ultimate fate? What is their bioavailability? How do they leave the body?

Unfortunately, compared to the amount of PK data that is collected for an FDA approved drug, there is nowhere near the amount of PK data for essential oil molecules.

But, that's ok. Why?

Because we now have millions of users who are actively using essential oils on a daily basis across the world. And the testimonies of these people can go a long way in drawing conclusions about the

PK of essential oil molecules. Also, the lack of any severe safety concerns among these millions of individuals demonstrates that these molecules are actively being cleared from our body.

What do we know about how fast essential oil molecules enter our bodies? To what extent do they reach the various cells in our body?

There are very limited studies in the literature regarding the absorption of essential oils into the different tissues of the body, and a moderate amount of research regarding their absorption from the skin and lungs into the bloodstream. So, based on this research, certain inferences can be made.

Let's take a look at a popular essential oil: Lavender. A study by Jager et al (1992) showed that after lavender oil was applied to the abdomen at a 2% dilution in peanut oil, linalool and linalyl acetate demonstrated peak concentrations in blood at approximately 20 minutes. After 90 minutes, the majority of the constituents were cleared from the blood.

Schuster et al. demonstrated that plasma levels of alpha- and beta- pinene, camphor, and careen, peak within 5 minutes after dermal application. Limonene peaked in about an hour.

So, it would appear that within 5-20 minutes that some constituents do indeed reach the blood stream following dermal application, while some constituents may take a bit longer. For example, Wang & Tso (2002) demonstrated that the plasma concentration of the constituent Bergapten peaked in 360 minutes after dermal application of Bergamot oil. The time for the constituent Thymol to reach peak concentration is approximately 120 minutes

(Kohlert et al 2002). The constituent from Peppermint oil can take up to 100 minutes to peak (Mascher et al 2001).

Many factors can vary the amount of time that it takes for the various constituents in the oil to reach the systemic blood stream. This process is subject to the biological variation common to humans. Age, skin condition, genetics, nutritional status, metabolism, epigenetics, etc, all can play a role in how readily skin takes up essential oil constituents into the blood stream. Also, constituent profile, dilution, and carrier system can all play a major role as well. There is limited data in the literature, and the data that is available appears to be sporadic---all due to the multiplicity of variables listed above.

Now, after these terpenoid and other classes of essential oil constituents are absorbed through the skin (or the lung tissue) and into the blood stream, where do they go? We know that terpenoid compounds are rapidly absorbed into different tissues, metabolized by the body through Phase I and Phase II reaction mechanisms, and ultimately excreted in the urine, feces, and in the form of CO_2 from the lungs. The metabolic fates and excretion mechanisms for each constituent is different. Generalization is not possible, because each constituent exhibits different metabolic kinetics and fates in the body.

The elimination profile of many essential oils is biphasic, meaning that the elimination concentration curve in plasma shows two different regions characterized by two different half-lives, inferring that there are two different major mechanisms controlling the elimination of the constituents. Kleinschmidt et al (1985) showed that intravenous injection of a mixture of terpenes exhibited an alpha phase half-life for 3-4 minutes, which suggests that the terpenes were rapidly cleared from the blood circulation into surrounding tissues. This is the first phase.

The second phase, called the beta phase, showed a half-life of 60 minutes, which is indicative of metabolism and excretion in a relatively short time frame —meaning that after the essential oils are absorbed into the tissues they are shortly thereafter metabolized and eliminated from the body.

These two processes are in competition with one another. First, the molecules are circulated throughout the blood and introduced to our tissues. Second, they are cleared from our tissues and recirculated into our blood stream, and metabolized by the liver and the kidneys. When these compounds are metabolized, they are oxidized and chemically transformed by our liver and kidneys into forms that can be readily eliminated through the body in the form of urine, feces, or CO_2 from the lungs. As they are eliminated in our urine, feces, and CO_2, the concentration of the molecules in our tissues begins to drop until all of the molecules are cleared from the body.

Before they are completely cleared, however, the molecules are distributed into the tissues of the body from transport across capillary walls into the various cells within tissues in which these capillaries are embedded.

It's important to realize that no experiment has ever been done to measure the amount of essential oil components that reach every organ, and every cell of the human body. The data on the pharmacokinetics of essential oils is quite limited when compared to the body of data that is available on other drug compounds.

However, it's important to note here that certain inferences can be made. First, most essential oil molecules are quite small, and quite lipophilic (meaning they like to be absorbed into biomolecular matrices that have a higher lipid concentration) This includes cell membranes and other compartments within the cell that are surrounding by lipid membranes and adipose tissue. All cells have a lipid membrane, so it is theoretically possible that essential molecules could diffuse into every cell membrane.

When you apply a drop of oil to your body, there is approximately 1,000,000 essential oil molecules for every cell in your body (the human body has about 60 trillion cells). Considering that essential oil molecules have been shown to cross the blood brain barrier, it's theoretically possible that every cell in your body could be exposed to more than one essential oil molecule.

However, practically, it's more complicated than that. For this to occur, every cell in your body would need to be reached by an essential oil molecule before the molecules are metabolized and excreted by the body. Certainly, there will be front-line cells that are first exposed to the essential oil molecules that readily absorb the molecules due to their lipophilic nature. Tissues that receive more blood flow are going to receive the lion's share of the essential oil molecules. Tissues that receive the largest portion of blood flow include the brain, kidneys, liver, lungs, and muscle tissue (only if the muscle tissue is in motion). As these tissues absorb these molecules, the plasma concentration declines, leaving less molecules for the secondary and tertiary tissues that receive less of the cardiac output.

Adipose tissue, for example, receives a relatively small amount of blood flow compared to these other tissues. But, due to the fact that adipose tissue is lipophilic, it will uptake what little of the essential oil molecules are delivered through circulation and store these molecules for a longer period of time before ultimately releasing them.

As discussed above, there is a competition. As the molecules are traveling through the systemic circulation, the body is metabolizing the molecules to eliminate them from the body. So, there is a competition between the rate at which the molecules are being introduced for cell absorption and the rate at which they are being eliminated from the body. This metabolic profile is different for each constituent in the oil.

So, at least theoretically, the essential oils could reach every cell in the human body. However, practically, that is probably not the case due to the complex dynamics at play governing the rate at which these molecules are absorbed, distributed, metabolized, and cleared. However, I would make a scientific guess that most (50-70%) of the cells in our body are being exposed to a larger or lesser degree to a profile of essential oil constituents contained within the original preparation. And that is just a reasonable guess.

If you're wanting to summarize this in simple terms, I would say the following:

> *Essential oil molecules are known to be rapidly taken up into the blood stream and to be distributed to many of the tissues throughout the body. Some constituents have been measured to be absorbed within 5 minutes, and some may take a few hours. Every essential oil and every person is different, but for the most part, the essential oil molecules are readily available to the tissues of our body.*

References

Kohlert, C., et al. "Bioavailability and pharmacokinetics of natural volatile terpenes in animals and humans." Planta medica 66.06 (2000): 495-505.

Jager, W., et al. "Percutaneous absorption of lavender oil from a massage oil." J Soc Cosmet Chem 43.1 (1992): 49-54.

Mascher, Hermann, Christian Kikuta, and Helmut Schiel. "Pharmacokinetics of menthol and carvone after administration of an enteric coated formulation containing peppermint oil and caraway oil." Arzneimittelforschung 51.06 (2001): 465-469.

Schuster, O., F. Haag, and H. Priester. "Transdermal absorption of terpenes from essential oils of Pinimenthol-S ointment." MEDIZINISCHE WELT 37.4 (1986): 100-102.

Wang, Lai-Hao, and Mey Tso. "Determination of 5-methoxypsoralen in human serum." Journal of pharmaceutical and biomedical analysis 30.3 (2002): 593-600.

Differences in Absorption Rates for Different Parts of the Body

Where is the best place on body to topically apply essential oils?

The answer is "we don't really know for certain," simply because detailed experimental studies in humans have not been conducted to compare the differences in absorption of essential oils when applied to different anatomical positions on the body. There is limited data on the percutaneous absorption of essential oils and a good deal of purified constituents, but no data that would allow a direct comparison between the different locations of the body.

So, we must look to what we do know. The good news is there is some comparative data on a limited number of other molecules that do allow us to draw conclusions about the permeability of different locations of the body to small, lipid soluble molecules.

A lot of this data was generated by Dr. Howard Maibach and Dr. Robert Feldmann at the Department of Dermatology at the University of California School of Medicine. There is other data by other researchers, but they generally corroborate the data I am going to discuss in this section, so this analysis will not be exhaustive.

The first data I would like to share with you is a study conducted by Maibach & Feldmann where they investigated the "regional variation" in the absorption of two pesticides, parathion and malathion. These are small organic molecules that are lipophilic, meaning that they like to partition into lipid matrices rather than water or aqueous based solutions. Generally, they prefer to absorb into substrates that are more fatty, because they, themselves are "lipophilic" or "lipid loving". It's important to remember that the constituents that make up essential oils are also small organic molecules that are more or less lipophilic, so this is a good system to use as a comparison to draw inferences from.

I took the data from the original paper's table, and graphed it so that you can see it visually. The horizontal axis is time in hours (not minutes). It's important to realize that these concentrations are indicative of the entire absorption and elimination process, because the concentration of each molecule (or metabolite) was measured in the urine. Nonetheless, we can use this data to infer the relative absorption rates of the molecules at different anatomical positions of the body.

The first graph is a time course of the excretion of parathion from urine after it was administered to certain anatomical positions on the skin, which are labeled in the graph:

Parathion Absorption Across Different Anatomic Regions (C14 Urinary Excretion)

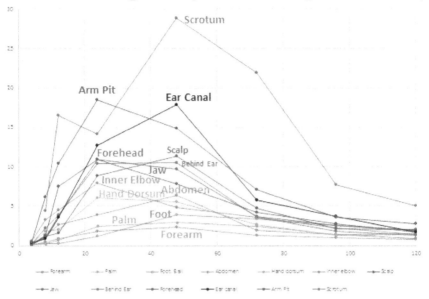

Time Course of Absorption of Pesticides From Different Locations of the Body

As you can see, the palm of the hand, and the ball of the foot were slightly better in terms of absorption than the forearm. The scrotum and the arm pit exhibited the highest absorption profiles, with the ear canal, scalp, forehead, behind the ear, and scalp falling in the middle between these two extremes.

So, as you can see, the urinary excretion of the pesticide parathion slowly rises and then peaks about 50 hours after administration to the bottom of the foot.

The previous data gave us a good indication of the rate of absorption. To calculate total dose – if you take this data and calculate the total absorption (by integrating the area under the curve and converting it into a % of total administered dose), you end up with the following graph:

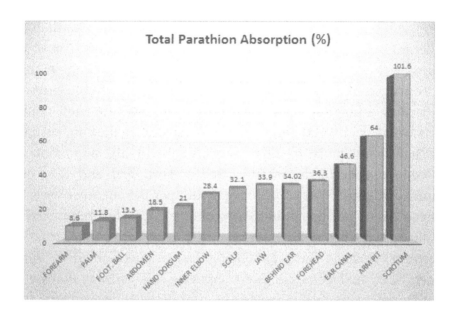

Total Dose Excreted Through Urine of Pesticides
Applied to Different Parts of the Body after 5 Days

The bottom of the foot exhibited about 14% absorption of externally applied parathion into systemic circulation and excretion. This was repeated for a subset of the anatomical locations for malathion, which is more hydrophobic (lipophilic) than parathion. The same general trend was noticed.

They also published data on the absorption of hydrocortisone, which is a steroid molecule that would mimic something like a sesquiterpene in terms of its chemical structure and size. The data was somewhat different, but generally the same.

You may have heard that the foot absorbs essential oil molecules because it has the highest density of "pores" per unit area than any other area of the body. There are actually no hair follicles/sebaceous pores on the sole of the feet; however, there is quite a large number of sweat glands, which could serve as access points to the egress of molecules into the epidermis. Sweat glands are not usually considered as efficient permeation points because they are designed for aqueous liquids to flow outward. There are approximately 250,000 sweat glands on the soles of both feet and they emit approximately ½ liter of water moisture per day. Because essential oil molecules are lipophilic (Hydrophobic), it is not reasonable to assume that they will enter via this pathway into circulation. However, perhaps there is some unknown mechanism by which essential oil molecules are able to traverse this pathway that we are simply not aware of due to the fact that detailed experiments have not been conducted. It's to be noted that these sweat ducts makeup something like 1–2% of the total surface area of the skin, so this is probably not the likely culprit.

Remember, no exhaustive data has been generated for the absorption of essential oil molecules across different locations of the body. When you have a complex mixture of 20–300 molecules, each with different polarities, chemical structures, sizes, and functional groups, there could be some type of coordinated synergistic mechanism that plays out which effectively permeabilizes the structural components of the epidermis, and allows the diffusion of essential oil molecules across the stratum corneum, through the epidermis, and into the underlying dermis. We saw this synergistic enhancement of permeation in the chapter on synergy with the example of Rose Oil.

The stratum corneum is the primary barrier to penetration, and it consists primarily of dead keratin-filled keratinocytes embedded in an extracellular lipid matrix. The foot epidermis possesses a very thick layer of stratum corneum (400-600 μM). Skin on the back, arms, abdomen, etc, is about 40-50 times thinner (8-15 μM). The stratum corneum of the underarm and groin is the thinnest. In the data discussed above, you can see that the absorption profile is inversely related to the thickness of the epidermis.

The lipids in the lipid matrix surrounding the keratinocytes are primarily sterols, other neutral lipids, and ceramides. Lipid soluble molecules (lipophilic molecules) can partition into this lipid matrix and diffuse in between cells (intracellularly).

Because essential oil molecules are lipid soluble, this is the assumed entrance pathway for molecules to penetrate the epidermis and enter into the lower dermal layer where they can then absorb through the capillary walls and enter systemic blood circulation.

My opinion is this: There is a large volume of testimonial data from essential oil users that is quite impressive when taken in its entirety, and I believe this information should not be dismissed or simply relegated as some mass placebo effect. Many people in the essential oil community attest to the observation that application of essential oils to the soles of feet more efficiently and more effectively imparts the bioactivity of the oil to the user. Until clinical trials are conducted that either confirm or deny these observations, I think the only honest scientific answer is we simply don't know.

One theory is that because the stratum corneum is so thick on the bottom of the feet, that this layer effectively acts like a "reservoir" that stores the essential oil molecules in the lipid matrix for extended durations and slowly releases them over time. In essence, the feet are a "time release" system that allows the essential oil molecules to diffuse into the blood stream slowly over time, and this extended release into the blood stream may have longer range biological effects that are not possible with "short bursts" that are normally associated with the skin layers that possess a much thinner stratum corneum. This slow release could continue for days.

This brings up another issue that I think is important to point out now. For some reason, I notice that people tend to be transfixed on the rate at which oils enter the body, as if the speed at which the essential oils peak in the system is somehow related to their efficacy. For an acute issue, like a headache, perhaps a fast rate is more favourable.

However, for a chronic issue, the rate at which the essential oil molecules are absorbed is an immaterial factor. The most important variable to consider for a chronic condition is "how long will the molecules be present in my system as a percentage of the day". If the molecules are rapidly absorbed and eliminated, then the molecules will only be present in the body for short bursts. The remaining time, the molecules are absent. In this type of situation, the person will need to apply many doses of essential oils around the clock.

What's more desirable for a chronic condition is a slow release of the essential oil molecules, so that there is a concentration of the oil molecules in the body at all times. For example, for chronic inflammation, high blood pressure, autoimmune disorders, and other chronic health diseases, it's better to have a low concentration of the oils present for a longer window of time than it is to have a high concentration of the molecules present for a shorter window of time.

So, for chronic health disorders, it may be advantageous to apply the oils to the bottom soles of your feet, which will act like a slow time-release capsule.

If you don't know which region of the body is the best, I encourage you to apply the same oil to different parts of the body, keeping all things constant. Allow a few days between experiments to ensure that the essential oils have completely cleared from your body tissues. Do you notice a difference? Does this difference only work with certain oils, or with all oils across the board?

References

Maibach, Howard I., et al. "Regional variation in percutaneous penetration in man." Archives of Environmental Health: An International Journal 23.3 (1971): 208-211

Feldmann, Robert J., and Howard I. Maibach. "Percutaneous penetration of hydrocortisone with urea." Archives of dermatology 109.1 (1974): 58-59.

The Blood Brain Barrier

Is it possible for essential oil molecules to cross the Blood-Brain-Barrier (BBB)?

The answer to this question is not definitive, but probable. It's probable that many essential oil molecules can readily traverse the blood brain barrier. No exhaustive study in humans has ever been undertaken to prove this point for the myriad of different molecules that are in essential oils, however there is good evidence that a large portion of the different essential oil molecules will make their way through the BBB into brain tissue. Several lines of evidence point to this.

The first line of evidence is the nature of the molecules that make up essential oils. They are of the right size and polarity to cross the blood-brain-barrier. Polarity is a measure of a molecule's degree of positive and negative charge distribution. More polar molecules tend to interact with more polar molecules, and less polar molecules tend to interact with less polar molecules. The scale that's used to measure non-polarity is related to the partition coefficient, LogP. LogP is a logarithmic scale that is a measure of a molecule's affinity for octanol (non-polar molecule) as compared to water (polar molecule), which is a way of measuring a molecule's lipophilicity (lipophilicity and non-polarity are similar terms). More non-polar/lipophilic compounds tend to like lipid/fatty type of environments and can easily cross through them.

Terpenes, one of the major classes of molecules in essential oils, fall on the LogP scale between 2-6. Non-polarity is a relative term, and it falls along a continuum, but generally LogP values in this range are considered to be non-polar molecules for the purposes of lipid transport across cellular membranes. What causes variability along this scale is the size of the molecule and the number of oxygen groups (and type of oxygen group). The presence of oxygen (such as a ketone, aldehyde, alcohol, carboxylic acid, or ether) lowers the LogP value because these functional groups are polar in nature and therefore lower the lipophilicity of the molecules.

Drugs that are designed to cross the blood brain barrier via the process of lipid transcellular diffusion fall in the sweet spot of LogP values of 1-3. Other drug molecules can cross the blood brain barrier via other mechanisms (receptor mediated transcytosis or active channels), so the LogP value doesn't play a role with this type of transport across the BBB. However, essential oil molecules are thought to use the lipid transcellular pathway, and so their LogP values fall into the range where this mechanism is active. Therefore, essential oil molecules fall in this range where transport across the blood brain barrier is possible.

Second, there is indirect evidence from mechanistic, neuropharmacological studies of the effects of essential oils in relevant in vivo models that demonstrate that the mechanism of action of the molecules are occurring in the central nervous system, and in particular, the brain. Measurable psychological effects that take place that go above and beyond the olfactory-limbic response indicate that the effects are primarily pharmacological, which mean the molecules are reaching the brain tissue to interact with certain receptors or other pathways. Limited clinical trials in the field of psychoaromatherapy are in line with this conclusion. As an example, a clinical trial in 20 volunteers demonstrated that cognitive performance was enhanced (both speed and accuracy for accomplishing cognitive tasks) for subjects that were exposed to rosemary aroma, and that the cognitive performance factors correlated with the plasma concentration of 1,8 cineole (a constituent found in Rosemary and other essential oils), with improved performance at higher concentrations [Moss & Oliver, 2012].

Third, ingestion of certain essential oils has shown identical effects to inhalation. If the effect was only observed during inhalation, it could be argued that the effect is only due to the stimulation of the olfactory-limbic system (i.e., the sense of smell affecting the limbic areas of the brain). However, Moss et al. 2010 report largely consistent effects for *Salvia officinalis* aroma compared with the effects of oral administration of extracts of these herbs as detailed by Scholey and colleagues [Scholey et al. 2008]. In addition, Kovar and colleagues assayed serum levels of 1,8-cineole, and recorded locomotor activity when rosemary oil was administered by inhalation or orally [Kovar et al. 1987]. The data showed that both the inhalation and oral administration of rosemary oil stimulated locomotor activity and that this was related to serum 1,8-cineole concentration.

Fourth, certain essential oil constituents have demonstrated the ability to cross the BBB in certain animal models. As an example, the constituent, Beta-elemene, which is a sesquiterpene found in essential oils, has demonstrated the ability to pass through the BBB in rat models, as it has been detected in rat brain tissue. Beta-Elemene is a sesquiterpene (C15 molecule) found in essential oils, and is prototypical of other similarly structured molecules found in essential oils (e.g., terpenes and terpenoids). Another study showed that linalool (a major constituent in essential oils) can be detected in mice at a high concentration in blood samples from the retrobulbar venous plexus after inhalation. Evaluation of (-)-linalool revealed a dose-dependent sedative effect on the central nervous system, including hypnotic, anticonvulsant, and hypothermic properties. In addition, in human trials, exposure to (-)-linalool resulted in cerebral blood flow reductions in the right superior temporal gyrus to insula, anterior cingulate cortex (ACC), and posterior ACC after inhalation. These effects point to pharmacological interaction with the central nervous system that is separate from the olfactory response.

Fifth, certain terpene molecules have been shown to modulate the activity of certain enzymes located in the brain that are involved in neuropharmacology, and this interaction is consistent with their observed physiological response. Orhan and colleagues reported that extracts of rosemary displayed significant inhibitory effects on both acetylcholinesterase (AChE) and butyrylcholinesterase enzymes, which are enzymes found in the central nervous system [Orhan et al. 2008]. Rosmarinic acid and ursolic acid, which are constituents found in rosemary, are inhibitors of AChE in vitro. In addition, 1,8-cineole, a major constituent found in many essential oils, possesses anti-AChE activity [Perry et al. 2000, 2003; Savelev et al. 2003]. It is believed that the neuropharmacological activity of certain essential oil constituents function via this anti-AChE pathway. Such activity is suggestive of the potential cognitive impact of essential oil molecules and forms the basis of pharmacological activity of a number of dementia treatments.

There are many "indirect" observations that suggest that essential oil molecules can cross the human BBB; however, an exhaustive study has not been performed in humans to directly prove this point for the thousands of different constituents that are found in essential oils. It's reasonable to assume that certain molecules will more readily cross this barrier than others, depending on their size and logP values as mentioned above.

References

Wu, Xue Shen, et al. "An investigation of the ability of elemene to pass through the blood-brain barrier and its effect on brain carcinomas." Journal of Pharmacy and Pharmacology 61.12 (2009): 1653-1656.

Nasel, C., et al. "Functional imaging of effects of fragrances on the human brain after prolonged inhalation." Chemical senses 19.4 (1994): 359-364.

Moss, Mark, and Lorraine Oliver. "Plasma 1, 8-cineole correlates with cognitive performance following exposure to rosemary essential oil aroma." Therapeutic advances in psychopharmacology 2.3 (2012): 103-113.

Sayowan, Winai, et al. "The effects of jasmine Oil inhalation on brain wave activies and emotions." Journal of Health Research 27.2 (2013): 73-77.

Sowndhararajan, Kandhasamy, and Songmun Kim. "Influence of fragrances on human psychophysiological activity: with special reference to human electroencephalographic response." Scientia pharmaceutica 84.4 (2016): 724-751.

Ota, Miho, et al. "(-)-Linalool influence on the cerebral blood flow in healthy male volunteers revealed by three-dimensional pseudo-continuous arterial spin labeling." Indian journal of psychiatry 59.2 (2017): 225.

Moss, L., Rouse, M., Wesnes, K. and Moss, M. (2010) Differential effects of the aromas of Salvia species on memory and mood. Hum Psychopharmacol Clin Exp 25: 388–396.

Scholey, A.B., Tildesley, N.T.J., Ballard, C.G., Wesnes, K.A., Tasker, A. et al. (2008) An extract of Salvia (sage) with anticholinesterase properties improves memory and attention in healthy older volunteers. Psychopharmacology 198:127–139

Kovar, K.A., Gropper, B., Friess, D. and Ammon, H.T.P. (1987) Blood levels of 1,8-cineole and locomotor activity of mice after inhalation and oral administration of rosemary oil. Planta Med 53: 315–319.

Orhan, I., Aslan, S., Kartal, M., Sener, B. and Baser, K.H.C. (2008) Inhibitory effect of Turkish Rosmarinus officinalis L. on acetylcholinesterase
and butyrylcholinesterase enzymes. Food Chem 108: 663–668.

Perry, N.S.L., Houghton, P., Theobald, A., Jenner, P. and Perry, E.K. (2000) In vitro inhibition of human erythrocyte acetylcholinesterase by Salvia lavandulaefolia essential oil and constituents terpenes. J Pharmacol 52: 895–902.

Perry, N.S.L., Bollen, C., Perry, E.K. and Bollard, C. (2003) Salvia for dementia therapy, review of pharmacological activity and pilot tolerability clinical trial. Pharmacol Biochem Behav 75: 651–658.

Savelev, S., Okello, E., Perry, N.S.L., Wilkins, R.M. and Perry, E.K. (2003) Synergistic and antagonistic interactions of anticholinesterase terpenoids in Salvia lavandulaefolia essential oil. Pharmacol Biochem Behav 75: 661–668

XIII. APPLICATION METHODS

What are the differences between the different application methods?

I n this chapter, we will briefly discuss the major differences between the different application methods: inhalation; ingestion; and topical application.

The table below is a summary of the different application methods to help explain the major differences between the three different methods of introducing essential oil molecules into your body.

	Organs Reached	Total Dose	Time of Absorption	Chemical Modification	Unique Advantages
Topically	all	low to high	Intermediate	Very Little	Local Treatment
Inhalation	all	very low	Fastest	Very Little	Stimulation of Limbic response
Ingestion	GI, kidneys, liver	low to high	Slowest	Yes	supporting GI and liver

Unfortunately, compared to the amount of pharmacokinetic (PK) data that is collected for an FDA approved drug, there is nowhere near the amount of PK data for essential oil molecules. We will now discuss each application method separately.

Ingestion

When you ingest a drug, nutrients, or even essential oil molecules, they enter your upper GI tract and then are absorbed in your upper small intestine. From there, they are transported through the Hepatic Portal Vein (HPV) where they are first introduced to the liver. The HPV collects venous blood from the spleen, gallbladder, pancreas, stomach, and intestines – and delivers this to the liver to detoxify any substances that may be harmful to the body before sending it to the systemic circulation. After leaving the liver, the blood travels to the heart via the inferior vena cava. The HPV supplies 75% of the liver's blood supply, where the other 25% originates from the hepatic artery.

When molecules that are foreign to the body (like drugs and essential oil molecules) pass through the liver, they are chemically transformed through a process called "first pass" metabolism. This lowers the bioavailability of many drugs, and in some cases, completely inactivates the drug molecule. This effect needs to be taken into account in the design of pharmaceutical drugs. In certain instances, the drugs that you consume are considered to be inactive "prodrugs" when you first ingest them, and then when they travel to your liver they are metabolized and then become "active" in your systemic circulation (e.g., codeine, morphine, salicin). Enzymes in the intestinal lumen, the intestinal walls, and in the microbiota living in your gut can also metabolize or chemically alter molecules before they are passed to your liver.

The purpose of this first pass metabolism is to chemically alter the molecule such that it is more readily secreted from your body through urine and feces.

With essential oils, there are a limited number of studies that have evaluated the vast number of metabolites that are produced after these molecules enter your liver and undergo first pass metabolism before being released into your systemic circulation. This is known to occur with essential oil molecules, but the degree to which this occurs for each of the tens of thousands of different essential oil constituents is currently unknown. It is "assumed" that this occurs for most of these molecules, and the various derivatives of each of these molecules is not well understood. Also, there is large genetic variability and enzyme expression levels among individuals with respect to the enzymes that perform these modifications in the liver and other tissues. Therefore, each individual is thought to metabolize essential oil molecules to varying degrees.

Therefore, when you ingest an essential oil, the molecules that are reaching the cells throughout your body are not in their original "native" format. They have been chemically altered in some way. A certain portion of them will be unmodified, but that % for each of the different essential oil constituents is not well understood, and again, would be a function of the genetic and physiological differences between individuals.

Does this mean that ingesting essential oils is bad? No. It just means that the effects are more unpredictable.

If you apply or inhale the molecules, they will not undergo this first pass metabolism through the liver before reaching the tissues of your body, but they will undergo this same metabolic fate as they eventually make their way to your liver and kidneys to be excreted from your body.

For these reasons, I recommend for most situations that oils be ingested for conditions that focus on the stomach, intestines, and liver. I make this recommendation because the essential oil molecules, for the most part, make their way to these organs in an unaltered state.

There may be isolated instances where someone should ingest an essential oil for an issue somewhere else in the body other than GI or liver. This is because in certain instances a clinical study may have evaluated the physiological effects on the body from ingestion of the oil and, therefore, the effects of these metabolites are already being taken into account. However, these studies will not address the genetic differences between individuals which may result in a different level of liver processing.

After essential oil molecules leave the liver, they are chemically modified. Please don't let that last statement intimidate or scare you. People have been ingesting oils for centuries, and practitioners prescribe them in this modality routinely. My point is that the effects may not be the same as you would expect if you apply them topically or via inhalation. Each application method has its own unique profile. In many instances you will find that the effects overlap, but you can't always assume that's going to be the case.

There is evidence that essential oils can enhance the absorption and overall bioavailability of micronutrients and vitamins being delivered into the body. For this reason, adding essential oils to supplements is beneficial.

In terms of total dose, the ingestion pathway offers a wide dosing window, from very small doses to very high doses that can be dangerous to your liver and the rest of your body. It is always wise to dilute in a carrier oil to ingest, and to remember the motto "more isn't necessarily better." Every molecule has a certain therapeutic bioactivity profile that governs the molecule's behaviour in your body based on dose. At lower concentrations there is a therapeutic advantage to the constituent's presence in your cells, and above a certain threshold concentration the effect can disappear and even turn towards toxicity at higher doses. Therefore, my advice is to take as little essential oil as possible, and to slowly work up in concentration until you notice the positive effect you are trying to achieve.   In many instances, 1-2 drops is more than enough for a given dose. It's also better to take very small doses more frequently, than it is to take large doses less frequently. This will make your liver very happy and will smooth out the concentration spike so that the effects last longer in your body.

With respect to timing – Ingestion is the slowest of the pathways. It can take 1-2 hours before the molecules go through your GI tract and enter your systemic circulation.

Topical Application

Topical application of essential oils is probably the best way to deliver essential molecules to the various tissues of your body. After the molecules penetrate your skin tissue, they directly enter your systemic circulation and then permeate the tissues and cells of your body. The molecules can even pass through the blood brain barrier.

When there is a complex mixture of 20-300 molecules, each with different polarities, chemical structures, sizes, and functional groups, a coordinated synergistic mechanism allows the molecules to effectively permeabilize the structural components of the epidermis, and allows the diffusion of essential oil molecules across the stratum corneum, through the epidermis, and into the underlying dermis.

The stratum corneum is the primary barrier to penetration, and it consists primarily of dead keratin-filled keratinocytes embedded in an extracellular lipid matrix. Lipids surround the dead keratinocytes. The lipids surrounding the keratinocytes are primarily sterols, other neutral lipids, and ceramides. Lipid soluble molecules (lipophilic molecules) can partition into this lipid matrix and diffuse in between cells (intracellularly). Because essential oil molecules are lipid soluble, this is the assumed entrance pathway for molecules to penetrate the epidermis and enter into the lower dermal layer where they can then absorb through the capillary walls and enter systemic blood circulation.

The foot epidermis possesses a very thick layer of stratum corneum (400-600 micrometers). Skin on the back, arms, abdomen, etc, is about 40-50 times thinner (8-15 micrometers). The stratum corneum of the underarm and groin is the thinnest. The time of the absorption profile is inversely related to the thickness of the epidermis. Therefore, the skin area where the stratum corneum is the thickest will provide the longest pathway into the bloodstream, and the skin area where the stratum corneum is the thinnest will provide the fastest route into the blood stream.

I find that many people get hung up too much on applying the oil where route of absorption is the fastest. Unless there is an acute condition where immediate relief is required, fastest isn't necessarily better. For chronic conditions, a slower time-release effect is more beneficial. In this instance, applying the oil where it is known that the delivery is slowed down over time (a thicker epidermal layer) is the better approach. The bottom of the foot is a great place for this type of time-release response.

Permeation through the skin occurs over a window of time that starts at 5 minutes, and can last for several hours depending on the constituent, the location of your body, and the amount of fat tissue present at the application site. For example, applying essential oils to the bottom of your feet will release essential oil molecules into your bloodstream for 24 hours or more.

Because the molecules enter your systemic circulation in their native state (not metabolized by your liver first), they can distribute to the various tissues and cells in your body in their original form. Eventually, they will be metabolized and excreted from your body, but your cell's first encounter with the molecule will be in its unaltered form. Because of this, the therapeutic activity of the oil is more predictable.

In terms of dosing, topical application can provide you with a very large dosing window. You can simply apply more oil to your skin to receive a higher total dose. However, I strongly recommend against applying oils "neat" (undiluted) for several reasons. First, you can develop sensitivities and allergic responses to oils if repeatedly applied to your skin in undiluted form.

Secondly, diluting the essential oil in a fixed oil before applying it to your skin can help deliver more of the lighter weight molecules into your circulation due to the reduced rate of evaporation of the more volatile, lighter molecules within the matrix of the fixed oil. Thirdly, diluting the essential oil enables you to apply the same dose of oil over a much larger surface area of skin, which improves overall absorption.

One of the unique benefits of topical application is it provides you with the ability to focus treatment on your body. You can certainly use this pathway to introduce the molecules to your systemic circulation which will reach all areas of your body, but you can also use this method to focus on your sore back, for example.

Inhalation

Inhalation is probably one of the most interesting aspects of essential oil usage, and probably one of the most misunderstood. First let's look at state, dosage, and timing, and then let's look at a unique aspect of breathing in essential oils.

After the essential oil molecules enter your lung tissue, they are not altered by metabolic processes; therefore, they enter your systemic circulation in their unaltered form, similar to topical application.

The lungs are extremely permeable to small lipophilic molecules, and even small peptides and larger proteins. The lungs are much more permeable to molecules than any other entry port into the body. The epithelial lining in the lung is about 0.2 micrometers in thickness in the alveoli. The entire cardiac output flows through the lung capillary network and perfuses its entire volume rapidly. Just as a point of reference, Xe-133 ventilation perfusion-lung scans are considered normal if a person's lungs clear the radioactive gas in less than 150 seconds.

This is the reason why the lung is the fastest entry vehicle for delivery of essential oil molecules into the body. Essential oil molecules are small (300 AMU or less) and lipophilic, so they are rapidly absorbed and do not "build up" in the lung tissue.

The average half-life for small, lipophilic molecules in the lung is ~1 minute. The half-life is defined as the amount of time required for half of the adsorbed dose to permeate and be cleared from the internal lung tissue.

The molecules in essential oils will not stick around for long in your lung tissue before they are absorbed and delivered to your entire body throughout your systemic circulation. For this reason, this is the fastest route of entry into your blood stream.

Even though this is the fastest route of entry, the total delivered dose is very limited. To highlight this, conceptualize what is ultimately occurring in this mode of application. Typically, you would dilute an oil into a water bath in a diffuser that dilutes the oil at least 10,000 fold. This water containing the diluted essential oil molecules is then diffused into the air in microdroplets over the course of 6 hours or more, into a room that is at least 50 to 60 thousand times larger than the total volume of the diffuser. Then, you inhale a very small % of that volume into your lungs in one breath. As you can see, very small amounts of the essential oils are reaching your blood stream in this method, but over a very long period of time.

So, what are the benefits of using this method, then?

Well, there is one effect that can't be replicated with any of the other methods of application, and that is the olfactory-limbic response.

When you breathe in essential oils, the molecules interact and stimulate the olfactory receptors lining the upper nasal cavity which, in turn, send electrical stimuli to the olfactory bulb and then the limbic region of your brain.

Humans have approximately 350 different olfactory receptors (protein molecules that are expressed on the surface of olfactory neurons and that can differentiate different chemical structures). Each olfactory receptor (OR) can recognize and bind to certain chemical structures. Each OR can bind to more than one chemical, and a chemical can bind to more than one OR. Therefore, each chemical in an odor can bind to more than one OR, which creates a unique signature or combination of OR's that are activated for that molecule. That pattern of uniquely activated OR's is what ultimately encodes odor identity.

If only three of the 350 OR's are activated for a given molecule, the number of unique OR combinatorial patterns could encode over 1 billion unique odors. Those OR's are spatially organized and mapped to the olfactory bulb through projected axons that terminate in glomuleri structures in the olfactory bulb. These glomuleri then project that code into the olfactory cortex in the brain. The brain then distinguishes if an odor is pleasant or unpleasant, which is qualitatively measured in a variable called the hedonic valence. Even a small change to a chemical structure (i.e., the entire bulk of the molecule remains the same except for one small functional group that changes), can change the hedonic valence from pleasant to unpleasant.

The olfactory bulb sends olfactory information to the limbic system deeper at the base of the brain. These limbic regions a role in emotion, memory, learning, and homeostasis of body functions. The orbitofrontal cortex, amygdala, hippocampus, thalamus, and olfactory bulb have many interconnections through olfactory cortex.

Functions of the Limbic System:
- Memory processing.
- Emotions
- Regulating eating, hunger and thirst
- Responding to pain and pleasure
- Controlling the autonomic nervous system – blood pressure, breathing, pulse, etc.

This pathway is only stimulated when the molecules enter your nasal cavity and interact with the olfactory receptors lining the upper nasal cavity. It is not induced via the molecules entering the systemic blood circulation.

This is the reason why aromatherapy can be so effective in helping to regulate someone's emotions, and in providing feelings of contentment and relaxation, as well as supporting the regulation other more basic autonomic functions of the body.

These are the major advantages of each of the different application methods, and the considerations to be aware of. This information will help you line up the proper approach with the therapeutic effect that is of interest in any given situation.

XIV. HOW TO CHOOSE THE RIGHT OIL

Where do I go from here?

W hen you have a certain problem, what's the best process to go through to choose the right oil? Or oil blend? Or to make your own blend? I'm sure all of us are familiar with the infographics/memes that have made the rounds that folks normally draw upon. Although these might be helpful to gain some initial insight, they are normally not verified for accuracy, and their origins remain elusive. To help guide you in your process, I'm giving you a structure to follow to help make the process easier, and, perhaps, more successful. Here is the process that I would use in making usage decisions.

1) First, make sure you have several good desk references/user guides or books for essential oil usage/aromatherapy. Life Science Publishing (www.discoverlsp.com) is a great resource to find great reference books.

It's good to keep several references so that you can compare with one another to determine if harmony or disagreement exists between the different sources for specific applications when they arise. There are many different references out there. The key is to keep several references written by unrelated authors with different backgrounds. If there are correlations or agreement, then this data becomes more believable. It's important to have more than one to provide comparative value. It's certainly possible that all references could get something wrong, or they may all be perpetuating folklore with no real substantiation, but the chance of that sort of thing is considerably minimized when multiple sources are in agreement.

It's important to understand that some usage application data is garnered through collective wisdom that is passed down, and it may not be possible to find peer-reviewed journal articles that corroborate the bioactivity of the oil. Many people would discard information that hasn't been corroborated by modern research, but I would implore anyone not to do this. Don't throw the baby out with the bathwater. There is value in understanding and considering the wisdom that has been passed down through the centuries that may have not been verified by peer-reviewed science quite yet. It's important to remember that, comparatively, there is very little research money out there for researchers to conduct research on natural products, so it's not surprising that a great deal of usage claims do not have a published research study to confirm its validity. A great deal of the information in the essential oil community relies on the wisdom passed down from other cultures, as well as current-day testimonials that have been accumulated.

2) When a particular issue arises, look it up in the references that you have on hand. Chances are that each reference will specify a different list of oils to try. Look for oils that are in agreement across the

multiple references and start with those as your short list. There may be one or two that are on top of each reference's list. If there are no commonalities, then choose the top one from each reference and place it on your short list. Make sure that you have the full Latin names of the species for each of the oils, and if applicable, the specific part of the plant from which the oil is derived.

3) Go to Google Scholar (scholar.google.com). Do not use google. Use Google Scholar. Google Scholar will search all research articles (including those in Pubmed and others, including patents). Type in the name of the species followed by "essential oil" and search out if any studies have been conducted that corroborate the recommendations made by your at-home references. You should also perform a search of the genus name without the species identifier. Also, you should perform a search for the common name of the essential oil. For example, if you were looking for information on Lavender, you should try these three search phrases:

- Lavandula angustifolia essential oil
- Lavandula essential oil
- Lavender essential oil

If the search turns up too many results for you to filter through, then try searching for the name of the plant in combination with the issue you're dealing with. For example, you could perform three searches for the following phrases

- Lavandula angustifolia anxiety
- Lavandula essential anxiety
- Lavender essential anxiety

Also, simply search for your "issue" along with the phrase "essential oil" This will help to add to your list if the oil wasn't mentioned in any of your references. For example, you could perform the following searches:

- Anxiety essential oil
- Anxiolytic essential oil

When you perform the search, you'll see a list of titles that you can click on to read the abstract. If you want to read the entire research paper, you may need to purchase the article, or in many instances now, the article is free. However, for most applications, you can glean enough information from just the title and the abstract to know if that oil is a good candidate to keep on your list.

By the way, this is a great skill set to develop. It's important that we all learn how to catch fish, and teach others to do the same.

It may take you 15-30 minutes to go through this process, but the information and the skill you will gain in doing makes this invested time well worth it! You will learn a great deal about what research is out there, what the current trends are, and you will begin to see the breadth and depth of what's known and what is not known. No desk reference has everything, and certainly, it's not current with the latest research. When you perform a search, you are observing the current state of affairs as it exists on the day you perform the search. Also, you will begin to understand how these essential oils work. Quite frequently, the research paper will go into the mechanism of how the essential oil is working at the cellular level. This is not information that is normally shared in a desk reference.

Also, as I will discuss below – your genetics, epigenetics, and the cause of your symptoms may be completely different than someone else. Performing these searches will help you to augment your list with other candidates that might be right for your biochemistry and situation.

Therefore, the desk reference is a great place to start to get your bearing. But don't rely solely on this information. Take the time to do the search, and see what you can learn! Become the master of your own health by obtaining a greater understanding.

4) If the references that you find in your search agree with your home desk reference library– great! Make a note of that so that you don't have to go through the same process, and the next time you look in your references, you can easily determine what information you've already vetted. If there's one oil that seems to be the best, and the rest really are secondary, then you know where you need to start.

5) If there are multiple oils that all look like they could work equally well, then rank them to the best of your ability. Given nothing else to hang your hat on, you could choose to rank them by what you have available in your home cabinet, or by cost, or by another other factor that you think is important (e.g. "I prefer the smell of this one").

Then, try the first oil on your list. Depending on your particular situation, you may choose to try the oil for a few days, a week, or a month, to get an accurate picture of its effects. Chronic situations require a longer time period to notice an effect when compared to an acute problem. So, if you've had chronic arthritis for 10 years, you may not feel the benefits for a few weeks of constant application. Also, keep in mind the difference between an oil that deals with the root cause as opposed to an oil that just covers up a symptom. For example, an essential oil with menthol in it may help to cover up the pain of arthritis and you will see an immediate relief. You may be fooled into thinking, "My arthritis is healed!" Not so. In a few hours your pain will return, and your arthritis hasn't improved any. In this situation, you should search for oils that can also help with the root cause: Inflammation and autoimmunity. These root causes will take a longer time to see a difference, but when they begin to take effect, the benefits will remain for a long period of time if you stop using the oils.

And this is why it's important to start learning how to do your own research. You can learn about the root causes of your problem, and then look for oils that deal with that root cause, rather than just focusing on relieving temporary symptoms. Make sense? The more you know, learn, and understand, the more you will be able to identify oils that start fixing the root cause.

During your trial, you should have some baseline parameter that you are measuring, and then look for changes in that parameter (positive, negative, or neutral) with respect to your initial baseline. If you notice a general trend of improvement over the time window you've defined, then you know that you have found something that works. If you see a negative effect or neutral effect, then move to the next oil on your list and repeat the process. For example, in this arthritis scenario, you should not only look at "is the pain gone", but you should also look at the appearance and mobility of your joint. Has the swelling and inflammation around the joint decreased? Do you have a greater range of motion? When I stop using the oil for a day, do these parameters persist? Considering your situation in this strategic way will help you know if you are truly seeing a benefit.

Make sure you use a journal and jot down your observations. Be precise so that if you look at your journal a year later, you can piece together the exact steps you took.

6) Blends – There's a few things about blends that I want to mention.

You should consider blends if it's a blend that you have already verified works, or if it's a blend that's been proven to work consistently by others, and you can verify that fact by group consensus. There's very little in terms of research literature that you can find on blends, so for the most part, Google Scholar and Pubmed won't help you much here. This is really the trickiest part. What's fact and what's fiction? What's real and what's simply the product of meme's or "group think" gone wild? Nine times out of ten it's almost impossible to track down the veracity of blend claims, and the blend's origins. Blends that are marketed by the big oil companies and that have been around a long time normally have some type of consensus in the aromatherapy community of efficacy, so I would consider those on a case-by-case basis. Even if there is widespread, general consensus regarding a blend (or even a single) I would still verify that the blend works for you! Genetically and biochemically, everybody is different. If you don't believe me, google the term "pharmacogenomics" and you'll be reading for years!

The error I see many people making is the error of the "mix it all together" approach. Basically, people make a list of every oil that's ever been shown to work, and then blend it all together with the idea that something ought to work in that mix. It's basically the philosophy of, "I don't want to miss out on anything and I want to maximize my chances of the oil working, so I'm going to put everything in there that even has a chance of working." I came across a meme that was shared by someone that basically prescribed a mixture of every single oil they could find, and then blends were blended into that whole mix on top of the singles! In my opinion, that has about a 2% chance of working! To see why, take this philosophy to its logical extreme---If you blend everything on the planet together, then it will do absolutely nothing because every constituent will be diluted as well as antagonizing one another in the "cellular interaction network" that I referred to in previous chapters. Too many chefs can spoil the stew.

In the absence of a well-known, or highly-vetted blend from a trusted source, I believe the best approach is to start out with a single. The less, the better, especially when you're attempting to piece a puzzle together regarding what oil is going to work for your situation. I'm not claiming that a blend won't work, or that a blend won't work better. My intent here is to get you used to the idea of thinking scientifically and breaking a problem down into simpler components. Adding a second or third oil into the mix will complicate the number of possibilities, and you may never focus in on the right combination. An oil is already a complex enough biochemical universe all to itself. For reasons I described in previous chapters, oils don't add together like numbers do. Biological systems don't work by the rules of algebra, unfortunately.

With those considerations in mind, if you want to experiment making your own blend, start with the process that I outline in 5). If that process yields two or more singles that barely-to-moderately work for your situation, then blend any two of them together (not three). Make three blend ratios. 1:3, 1:1, and 3:1. Trial each one for the time window that you initially prescribed and note the change from baseline. There's a possibility that two of the low-to moderately functioning oils will work together synergistically to improve efficacy, but there is no guarantee. Again, this is not something that is predictable with 100% confidence.

Functional Group Theory – There is a prevailing theory in the aromatherapy community that is based on predicting the activity of an oil by the relative presence of certain classes of chemical functional groups. What are functional groups? They are smaller chemical groups that are attached to another larger core chemical structure –chemical groups like Aldehydes, Ketones, Carboxylic Acids, Ethers, and Alcohols are considered functional groups.

In functional group theory, it's assumed that all essential oil molecules that have an alcohol group do X, and all essential oil molecules that have an aldehyde group do Y, so on and so forth. The only problem with this approach is that it is fundamentally flawed. Two different constituents, each possessing an alcohol group (-OH), could have entirely different bioactivity profiles. Why? Because constituents exert their effects by binding to specific biological targets, like protein molecules in our cells. The constituents fit into specific geometric cavities on the surface of proteins and other biomolecules, and this binding compatibility is based on a key-and-lock type of fit. The functional group (like the alcohol group) represents only a small portion of the complete chemical geometry of the constituent.

As an analogy, the functional group would be equivalent to one small tooth on a key that has 78 teeth. It would be like claiming that you could predict the lock that a specific key would fit into by looking at just one of the teeth on the key, and then assume that the key will fit every other lock that accepts that one tooth!!! It's the entire pattern and geometry of teeth that matter. In the same way, it's the entire chemical structure of the constituent that matters, not the little functional group that's protruding off a certain portion of the molecule. The reason I bring this up is because a lot of the blends that are developed are based on the assumption from functional group theory. "Use this oil, because it has 17% aldehyde content and aldehydes do X".

To understand why this doesn't work, you need to have a basic understanding of not only chemistry, but molecular biology. When you go through my classes, you'll quickly see why this approach doesn't work. The same reasoning holds true for entire classes of molecules, like monoterpenes, and diterpenes, and sesquiterpenes, etc. You can't predict the activity of an entire class of molecules simply because humans have found a way to classify them by the number of carbons that make up their backbone. If that were the case, you could predict the activity of a drug molecule simply by counting up the number of carbon atoms it contains. Unfortunately, many blends have been made with this philosophy.

So, those are some tips on how to choose the right oil, and maybe even more importantly, how NOT to choose an oil. I hope this information is helpful to you!

So, there you go. Follow those steps above to find the right oil for your given situation. Keep good notes and records in an easy-to-find place. The next time you are presented with a situation, the research is already done. You may choose to do another quick search online to see if any new research has been published, but for the most part, your prior research will translate into the future and will make your job easier and you build up a knowledge base.

Just think, you will be able to help others with the knowledge base that you accumulate, and you will be able to help people by communicating to them your experience. There is nothing more powerful than sharing with someone your experience and being able to back that up with research.

The next obvious question is: "Why would one oil work for my friend Sally, but it didn't work for me when I used it for the same issue?

That's the subject of the next chapter.

XV. WHY DOESN'T THIS OIL WORK FOR ME?

Everyone is the same, but different

Have you ever been frustrated to find that after trying an essential oil, you didn't notice any benefit? Especially when it's an oil that every book and person you spoke with recommended for that particular issue? Or, perhaps, you shared an oil that worked for you for a particular situation with someone else, and they didn't have the same experience. You are certainly not alone. This is a common question, and its answer is a bit complex. There are many reasons why this may be so, and I'm going to answer this as simply as I know how.

First off, the therapeutic profile of an oil is tied directly to the synergistic interactions that take place among the host of constituents that make up the oil. Synergy is defined as when the sum of the parts is greater than the sum of the individual components. Please brush up on this topic in the previous chapters of this book. This happens more often than not with essential oils. In fact, there are examples where certain constituents by themselves have no therapeutic potential on their own accord, but when combined with another constituent in the proper ratio, a completely new activity manifests itself that is not exhibited by either constituent alone. In many cases these constituents that activate the synergistic potential of the other components are considered trace components, meaning that they are found in relatively small concentrations when compared to the other constituents. Some constituents that are necessary to activate the potential of the oil may only make up less than 0.1% of the oil.

Now, what factors dictate the composition of the oil? The composition of the oil is a direct function of a long sequential list of factors, processing steps, and quality control techniques. Just to highlight some of those factors: seed chemotype, soil nutrient profile, weather conditions, farming practices, harvest time (month, day, and time of day), distillation conditions (geometry of distiller, temperature, pressure, time, and materials), and quality control measurements (GCMS, IRMS, HPLC, Chiral GC) and appropriate libraries (chemical libraries and software libraries) – all play a role in dictating the final composition of the oil. If any of these factors are not right, then the oil may be missing key trace components that are necessary to activate the synergistic power inherent in the oil. All of the "big players" may be in the oil, but if one or more trace components are not present, then the oil's therapeutic profile could be severely debilitated. I go over all these factors in my book, "Innoilvation." You can get this book at www.StarFishScents.com.

This is why a process that defines a critical pathway for producing a particular oil is necessary to result in an oil that has all of the necessary components to do its work. And this is why it's very important to consider the company when using essential oils. The company should have control of the process from the time the seed goes in the ground, to the time the bottle is sealed, and every step in between. They should also have the proper chemical libraries and analytical expertise to identify the constituents in the oil. If some of those are missing, then the game completely changes. It's not enough to get "most of it right." All of it has to be right.

If you find that an oil isn't working for you, then the first the thing I would take a hard look at is the source and quality control standards associated with the company that produces that oil. If those are questionable or undefined, then I would suspect that as the main reason why the oil may not be working for you.

Second, everyone's bodies are different. There are three main factors that separate all of us:

1) Our primary Genetic Code
2) Our Epigenetic Code
3) Our Physiological Status

Let's handle the genetic code first. Each one of us have 3 billion letters residing in the main program that operates our body —DNA. Although most of that genetic code is similar from person to person, we all have differences when you line up that code side by side. There are approximately 4 million "single nucleotide polymorphism" (SNPs) among humans. A SNP is a single letter in the DNA that varies when you compare different people. That means that the genetic code at each one of those sites in the DNA is different from person to person. In addition, there are structural variants in the genetic code. All told, about 24 million of the 3 billion letters (0.8%) in the genetic code can differ from individual to individual. That's part of what makes us all unique.

Because the core genetic program is different from person to person, the proteins, and the expression levels of our proteins, are somewhat different. Remember what essential oil molecules do? They interact with proteins in the "Cellular Interaction Network." If the amount of each protein is different from person to person, then the interactions could also be somewhat different. The effects may not completely different, but there will be some differences. Therefore, the same constituents may interact somewhat differently in your body as they do in someone else's body. Bottom line, an oil that works for you for a certain condition may not work exactly the same for someone else for the same condition.

Now, let's handle the epigenetic code. The extent and significance of the epigenetic code is really the product of recent revelations. No scientist ever imagined that the epigenetic code would play as large a role in differentiating individuals as they are discovering. In fact, many scientists believe that the epigenetic code differentiates us more as individuals than the core genetic program. What is it? The epigenetic code is basically another layer of information that rides along the top of the DNA. It is in the form of chemical modifications to the chromosomes. These chemical modifications are the product of our life experiences. Stress, trauma, and even the entire history of the food we eat and the toxins that we have been exposed to affects the epigenetic code. And the worst part? Scientists are now beginning to understand that the epigenetic code can be passed on to our children, and that we can inherit certain aspects of it from our parents, grandparents, and great-grandparents. In other words, our experiences can affect our children more than the core genetic code. The epigenetic code can affect expression levels of each protein, and the precise structure of each protein.

Why is this important? Well, if you're using an essential oil and it works for you for a certain condition, you can't automatically assume that it will work for your IDENTICAL TWIN!!! Your identical twin's epigenetic code will differ from yours because their experiences are different.

Now, let's handle the third point – the status of our physiology. Even with people with the same genetic code and similar epigenetic codes, the make-up of their bodies and their current level of health could be dramatically different. One person may have more fat tissue than another. One may have a different spectrum of toxins residing in their adipose tissue depending on what they've been exposed to. One exercises more than another. One drinks more water than another. One person takes nutrients each day, and the other doesn't. The list of different habits and exposure variants are limitless, and each of those factors affects the physiology of our body. And to a certain extent, that physiology can affect how you respond to a certain essential oil.

Have you ever wondered why pharmaceutical drugs don't work the same for every person? Did you ever catch a glimpse of a clinical trial that makes the claim that the drug had a certain effect in only a certain percentage of the population? That's because of each of the three factors I mention above. Pharmacogenomics is built around this concept that drugs need to be tailored to our specific genetics. Remember, western medicine is built on the foundation of one molecule being introduced into our body. If one molecule can find itself in a universe of differences when introduced into our bodies, how much more so will the 100–300 constituents in an essential oil?

Our genetics and epigenetics also affect the vast repertoire of metabolizing enzymes that are found in our liver – both their expression levels and precise structure. Therefore, we will all metabolize oils somewhat differently. Our bodies might inactivate or activate certain constituents differently than someone else, and with a different kinetic profile (more slowly or more rapidly than someone else).

This is why I believe the best approach to essential oil usage is to experiment. It's good to have reference books, guides, usage groups, and PubMed articles to give us a place to start, as I describe in detail in the previous chapter. A large majority of the time, this process will work without too many surprises. So, start there. If that first iteration doesn't work for some reason, try oils that are lower down in the priority list. Some of those outlying oils may be exactly what your body needs. Learn to experiment and to discover this information for yourself. I think you will have greater success if you follow this approach.

What about the effect of Dose?

Because our bodies are different, the dose profile may be different between individuals as well. In addition, an oil may not work for you because you are applying too little, or even too much! This is one of those questions that is important to get right. We all know the old adage "Too much of a good thing can be bad". The same is true with essential oils.

This is difficult for many people to understand. The common misconception is that if something is good, then more of it should be even better. And I see many people applying this philosophy to how they use essential oils. Essential oils are not food. But even eating too much broccoli can be bad for you if that's what your entire diet consists of. Too much water can kill you.

I'm going to show you biochemical proof that there is an optimal dose window that we should all pay very close attention to. If you exceed the window, you can completely nullify the positive effects of the essential oil, and taken too far, you can begin to show signs of toxicity.

In the graph below, I show you the results of a study that was performed on cells that help build our bone tissue.

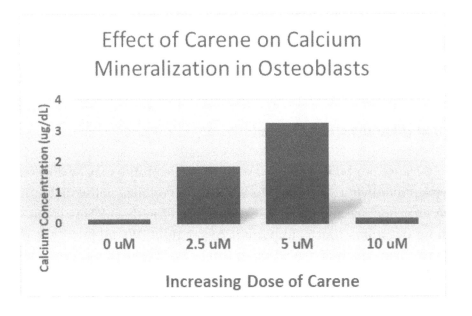

The types of cells that this experiment was performed on are called osteoblasts. Studies have shown that a constituent like 3–carene (which is found in essential oils) can induce anabolic like activity in osteoblasts which causes them to build bone tissue. In the figure above, you can see that they increased the concentration of 3-carene that was floating around in the media of the bone cells. You can see that there is a build-up of calcium upon introduction of 3-carene, meaning that these cells were now mineralizing calcium- which is what we all want for healthy bones! Especially if we are suffering from osteoporosis.

But notice what happens when they increase the 3-carene level to 10 uM. The calcium levels completely drop back to the level that would have been realized if the cells were not exposed to 3-carene at all!

There is an optimal concentration for this effect to take place. This type of "inverted U" is seen repeatedly in pharmacology. There is an optimal concentration for just about every compound --too much and the effect vanishes.

So, how much of any essential oil should you take? That's a great question with no simple answer. Everyone is different for the reasons I outlined in this chapter.

So, what do you do? Start small. If you've been using essential oils for a long time, perhaps you're frustrated because you do not notice a difference. Where most people would tell you to try more, I am going to tell you to try less. In fact, use the lowest amount where you start to notice a significant effect. Learn your body chemistry. Experiment with different dilution ratios, and find out what works for you! Keep good records/logs so that you can track the optimal dose that works for your body chemistry.

This is one reason why the foot might be a great place to apply essential oils for certain situations. As discussed in a previous chapter, the foot acts as a time-release system, lowering the concentration of the essential oil molecules in our body while spreading the dose out over a longer period of time. This type of dose profile can help to regulate the dose to a more consistent, lower level, rather than a rapid spike where the dose fluctuates wildly over a short period of time. That's not to say that a rapid, short dose might be what you need for a certain situation. For example, a burn or cut will benefit from a more aggressive approach.

In summary, everyone is different. Don't let that discourage you, though. For the most part, the same oils will work in most people. However, there will be instances where that's not the case, and now you know why and what to try in that scenario.

References

Jeong, Jong-Geun, et al. "Low concentration of 3-carene stimulates the differentiation of mouse osteoblastic MC3T3-E1 subclone 4 cells." Phytotherapy research 22.1 (2008): 18-22.